Periodontal Medicine – A Window on the Body

Periodontal Medicine
A Window on the Body

By
Iain L C Chapple
John Hamburger

Editor-in-Chief: Nairn H F Wilson
Editor Periodontology: Iain L C Chapple

Quintessence Publishing Co. Ltd.
London, Berlin, Chicago, Paris, Milan, Barcelona, Istanbul,
São Paulo, Tokyo, New Delhi, Moscow, Prague, Warsaw

British Library Cataloguing-in Publication Data

Chapple, Iain L. (Iain Leslie)
  Periodontal medecine; a window on the body. – (Quintessentials of dental practice; 43/44.
  Periodontology; 5)
  1. Periodontics
  I. Title II. Hamburger, John
  617.6´32

ISBN-10: 1850970793

ISBN 1-85097-079-3

This text is dedicated to my second daughter,
Natasha Sophie Chapple, born 17th August 2004

Iain L C Chapple

Foreword

'Periodontal Medicine' is an intriguing title for the latest addition to the rapidly expanding, widely acclaimed *Quintessentials in Dental Practice* series. Building on differential diagnoses for periodontal manifestations of systemic diseases and the role of relevant special investigations, this compact text of immediate practical relevance provides a unique consideration of gingival colour changes, enlargements, ulcerations and recession, not to forget a concluding miscellany of other gingival lesions.

This book is novel and therefore another pleasing first for the timely *Quintessentials in Dental Practice* series. In common with all the other volumes in the Series, 'Periodontal Medicine' can be read and easily digested over a matter of a few hours. This time will be well spent, with a lasting legacy of enhanced insight and understanding of conditions of the periodontium. Once read, this book should not be put on a shelf to gather dust. In contrast, it should become a well-used aide-memoire to keep to hand in everyday clinical practice. Excellent clinical pictures generously illustrate the carefully crafted text, making this attractive volume another jewel in the Quintessentials crown. The authors are to be congratulated on the special qualities of this book.

Nairn Wilson
Editor-in-Chief

Preface

Periodontal Medicine is a term used for different purposes in different parts of the world. In North America, it relates to the study of the dynamic relationship between periodontal diseases and systemic conditions, such as cardiovascular and cerebrovascular disease, pre-term labour and low-birth-weight babies, diabetes mellitus, osteoporosis and disorders of the respiratory tract. Such studies investigate the peripheral impacts of periodontal inflammation on systemic health and also the influence of systemic diseases on the progression of chronic periodontitis, such as type 2 diabetes mellitus, where evidence exists for a bi-directional relationship with periodontitis. However, in the UK and parts of Europe 'periodontal medicine' is a term used to describe the periodontal (and gingival) manifestations of medical conditions. This includes their investigation, diagnosis and therapeutic management and how management of the oral condition integrates with the patient's medical management as part of a holistic approach within defined care pathways. My own periodontal practice (ILC) relies heavily upon close working relationships with medical and surgical colleagues and joint patient management with bi-directional feedback, discussion and decision-making. In order of frequency, joint care is provided with Oral Medicine, Dermatology, Genito-Urinary Medicine, Cardiology, Clinical Immunology, Paediatric Medicine, Nephrology, Haematology, Gastroenterology, Geriatric Medicine, Ear/Nose/Throat and Maxillofacial Surgery.

This text therefore aims to provide the reader with an illustrated approach to managing the oral consequences of systemic diseases that present within and around the periodontal tissues. We have used the clinical appearance of the lesions as the starting point for discussion so that practitioners can follow a logical step-wise approach to differential and definitive diagnosis and subsequent management, either themselves, or through referral for secondary care. Some lesions are extremely common and others rare, and therefore each chapter tabulates the lesions that fall within its boundaries at the beginning of the chapter, but only discusses in detail the more common conditions. The final chapter discusses the less common non-plaque-induced conditions outwith their natural visual grouping.

Outcomes of Reading This Text

This text will not deal with plaque-induced periodontal conditions, but will focus on non-plaque-induced lesions and their management. It is hoped that having read this text the reader will be able to:

- Recognise the broader scope of clinical periodontology and the importance of medical management in addition to the traditional surgical focus of the discipline.
- Recognise the importance of close liaison with colleagues in oral medicine and pathology.
- Take a systematic approach to medical history-taking that extends routine questions into certain relevant areas of enquiry that involve the body in general.
- Examine oral lesions systematically and use the findings of specific features of the lesion and associated signs and symptoms, to start formulating differential diagnoses.
- Identify non-periodontal sites that may be affected by the presenting condition and what features to note at those sites.
- Return to the verbal enquiry and identify relevant follow-up questions that may further clarify the findings of the clinical examination – re-focus the history.
- Understand when additional clinical investigations are indicated, which are appropriate and how to perform them.
- Be able to interpret the findings of routine clinical investigations (e.g. blood test results) and develop a sense of the potential implications for the patient.
- Advise the patient about the aetiology of non-plaque-induced periodontal lesions.
- Identify the need to refer for advice or treatment by dental or medical specialists.
- Understand how the routine treatment he or she provides may impact, either positively or negatively, upon the condition.
- Identify a range of therapeutic options for the patient and understand the need for regular review and re-appraisal of the condition as appropriate.

Iain L C Chapple
John Hamburger

Acknowledgements

Iain Chapple wishes to thank his wife Liz and daughters Jessica and Natasha for their unconditional support and forbearance during the preparation of this book.

John Hamburger would like to thank his wife Ros and daughter Rachel for all their support and understanding during the preparation of this book.

The authors would also like to thank their colleagues within Periodontology and Oral Medicine. In particular Mrs Lorraine Williams and her staff who have approached the changes of the last 10-years so positively with enthusiasm, vigour and open minds. In addition, we are most grateful to our colleagues across a diverse range of medical specialties who offered their valued advice generously during the multidisciplinary management of our more complex patients.

We are indebted to Ms Jan Poller for her skillful proof reading of the manuscript and to Mr Michael Sharland and Ms Marina Tipton (Multi-media Services, Birmingham Dental School), Mr Paul England and Mr Jason Pike and colleagues (Clinical Illustration, Birmingham Dental Hospital). Thanks are also due to Mrs A Richards for permission to use Fig 2-2; Drs Barboza and Cunha and the British Dental Journal for the use of Fig 5-13; to Mr Mo Sandhar for the use of Fig 11-11; Mr D Glenwright for Figs 1-6, 1-10, 5-1, 5-8, 5-9, 5-15, 5-18, 10-10 and 10-21; Dr M Saxby for Figs 6-13a and b, Mr A Roberts for Figs 10-18 and 10-19; Mr M Milward for Fig 10-22; Mr J Rout for Figs 11-5a-e, 11-11, 11-12, 11-14, 11-15, 11-16, 11-18, 11-19, 11-24, 11-27a and b, 11-28, 11-29, 11-30, 11-31 and 11-32; Professor P Heasman for Figs 11-25a and b and Professor R Seymour for use of Fig 6-22.

Contents

Chapter 1
Establishing a Differential Diagnosis for Periodontal Manifestations of Systemic Diseases

Aim

This chapter aims to provide the reader with a step-by-step guide to history-taking, examination and further investigation of non-plaque-induced lesions that arise within the periodontal tissues, including the free and/or attached gingiva and associated oral mucosa, to help establish a differential diagnosis.

Outcome

Having read this chapter the reader should appreciate the need for a forensic and systematic approach to establish differential diagnoses for oral and medical conditions that manifest within the periodontal and associated tissues.

Terminology

A variety of clinical, procedural and pathological terms and descriptors are used throughout this chapter, and Table 1-1 defines these by category.

Guiding Principles Behind Establishing a Diagnosis

The sub-headings used in the following section are those classically recommended for use in clinical practice and thus are standard procedures.

In periodontal medicine, the 'history' has a unique temporal relationship with the other diagnostic stages, because it should continue throughout the consultation process, i.e. never hesitate to return to and refine the history in the light of each new piece of information gathered.

The Diagnostic Pathway

The Complaint
The complaint is information that must be provided by and recorded in the patient's own words. It is important when the complaint involves a symp-

Table 1-1 **Terminology Used in Periodontal and Oral Medicine/Pathology**

Context	Terminology	Definition
Clinical presentation or procedure	Symptom	Something the patient is experiencing or complaining of as a consequence of their condition.
	Sign	Something the clinician detects (visual, tactile or olfactory) that may help inform the diagnosis.
	Biopsy	Acquisition of human cells or tissues to aid diagnosis.
	Incisional biopsy	A biopsy involving partial removal of the lesion. This may be performed when malignancy is suspected and complete excision of the lesion would result in loss of key surgical landmarks.
	Excisional biopsy	A biopsy involving complete removal of the lesion.
	Fine needle biopsy /aspirate	Cells acquired using a fine cutting biopsy needle to obtain diagnostic material from within a lesion whose location or nature is such that surgical management should be delayed until microscopic diagnostic information is available.

Context	Terminology	Definition
	Broad needle biopsy	Tissue acquired using a broad cutting biopsy needle. The purpose is to acquire diagnostic material from within a lesion whose location or nature is such that surgical management should be delayed until microscopic diagnostic information is available. In addition, it is believed that acquisition of small numbers of cells may be of limited/no benefit to the pathologist.
	Swab	Use of a soft material (e.g. cotton pellet) to obtain infective material for culture and subsequent identification and testing (e.g. for antibiotic sensitivity) following culture.
	Smear	Use of a solid/sharp instrument to scrape away cells for microscopic examination.
	Cytology	Examination of individual cells (human or microbial) by microscopy, with or without special stains.
	Differential diagnosis	A list of possible diagnoses, ranked in order of the most likely to the least likely.
	Presumptive (working) diagnosis	A clinical diagnosis made in the absence of confirmatory information from additional clinical investigations and upon which therapy is based.

Context	Terminology	Definition
	Definitive diagnosis	The working and most likely diagnosis upon which therapeutic strategies are based.
Lesions and lesion descriptors	Ulcer	A breach in the epithelium to expose the underlying connective tissue.
	Erosion	A partial breach in the continuity of an epithelial surface, which does not expose underlying connective tissue.
	Fissure	A narrow crack or slit (usually describes an ulcer shape).
	Vesicle	A small (<0.5cm) fluid filled lesion (not pus)
	Bulla	A larger (>0.5cm) fluid filled swelling (not pus)
	Blister	A fluid filled swelling (not pus)
	Papule	Raised lesion (<1.0cm diameter)
	Macule	Flat lesion (<1.0cm diameter)
	Nodule	Raised lesion (>1.0cm diameter)
	Pedunculated	Lesion is borne/carried on a stalk/stem

Context	Terminology	Definition
	Sessile	Lesion is borne on a broad/flat base
	Sinus	A hole communicating a body cavity with the external environment
	Sinus tract	An epithelial lined tunnel linking an internal body cavity with the external environment
	Fistula	A communication between two body cavities
	Tumour	A neoplasm is an abnormal mass of tissue, the growth of which is uncoordinated with that of normal tissues, and that persists in the same excessive manner after the cessation of the stimulus which evoked the change
	Granuloma	A well-defined accumulation of modified macrophages (epithelioid cells), surrounded by lymphocytes and often with multinucleated giant cells.
	Epulis	A benign localised swelling of the gingiva usually affecting the interdental papilla
	Cyst	A pathological fluid filled (not pus) cavity.

Context	Terminology	Definition
Pathological terms or descriptors	Atrophic	Thinning of a tissue.
	Hyperplasia	An increase in the size of a tissue due to an increase in the number of its constituent cells.
	Hypertrophy	An increase in the size of a tissue due to an increase in the size of its constituent cells.
	Overgrowth	An increase in the size of a tissue due to an increase in the size and/or number of constituent cells and/or extracellular matrix components.
	Dysplasia	Disturbance in the normal maturation of a tissue.
	Anaplasia	Lack of differentiation of a tissue, characteristic of some tumour cells.
	Acantholysis	Separation of epithelial cells within the stratum spinosum.
	Acanthosis	An increase in thickness of the stratum spinosum.
	Leukoplakia	An adherent white patch or plaque that cannot be characterised clinically or pathologically as any other lesion (WHO).

Context	Terminology	Definition
	Erythroplakia	A bright red velvety plaque that cannot be characterised clinically or pathologically as any other recognisable condition (WHO).
	Hyperkeratosis	Excess deposition/formation of keratin within the stratum corneum of epithelium.
	Oedema	The collection of inflammatory fluid exudate within a tissue or body cavity.
	Angioedema	A diffuse oedematous swelling that may develop rapidly often involving the facial tissues and frequently, but not universally, results from a hypersensitivity reaction.

tom such as 'pain' or 'soreness' to clarify the exact details of that complaint, e.g.:
- Character?
- Intensity/severity?
- Location?
- Spread?
- Associated signs or symptoms?
- Similar lesions elsewhere on the body?

The History of the Complaint

The history of the complaint often holds the key to its diagnosis. For example, the appearance of the lesion or symptoms may be subsequent to the patient commencing new medication, implying a potential aetiological role for that medication. For an abscess that is of pulpal origin, any swelling may present after an episode of dental pain, whereas with an abscess of periodontal origin the swelling often precedes the development of pain; temporal issues are important. Other key issues to explore include:
- Onset?
- Duration?
- Aggravating factors?
- Relieving factors?
- Associated symptoms?
- Current status (i.e. improving or becoming worse?)
- Previous episodes?

Often by careful and detailed history taking it is possible to form a provisional diagnosis before even examining the subject, (but be wary of this approach to ensure you do not become biased). Some patients are good historians and others poor. It is important to record historical findings in a logical and succinct manner, which may be a challenge in the latter type of patient. It is good practice to return to a more focussed history after the clinical examination has provided pointers towards further questions which may help clarify the diagnosis.

The Medical History

A thorough medical history is essential and the process should be a staged one. Some of the issues highlighted below impact upon patient management and others are important in establishing a diagnosis. Key systems to explore would be:
1. *Cardiovascular system* – including cardiac murmurs, a history of rheumatic fever or infective endocarditis, blood pressure, cardiac surgery.

2. *The respiratory system* – including evidence of atopic disease e.g. metal allergies, allergies to drugs, asthma, chronic obstructive airway disease or granulomatous conditions such as sarcoidosis, T.B.

3. *The central and peripheral nervous systems* – a history of epilepsy, fitting, blackouts, neurological or neuropathology.

4. *The musculoskeletal system* – diseases or disorders of bone or muscle, connective tissue diseases.

5. *The vascular system* – evidence of haemorrhagic disease (e.g. idiopathic thrombocytopenic purpura – ITP), bruising, clotting disorders or disorders of the lympho-reticular system.

6. *Endocrine problems* – diabetes, thyroid or sex hormone/androgen disorders, including adrenal function. If diabetic, how well controlled is the diabetes? How often does the patient check their glucose levels? Do they know their last HBA1C level? A well-informed and health-conscious diabetic should know their most recent HbA1C level (see Book 1 of this series, Chapple and Gilbert).

7. *Renal or urinary tract* problems may be relevant to diagnosis or management. For example, patients who have been or are currently suffering from chronic renal failure may present issues surrounding:
    *   Calcification of cardiac valvular tissue secondary to chronic hypercalcaemia (need for antibiotic prophylaxis).
    *   Metabolism of drugs that may be considered for their oral disease.
    *   Hypertension (e.g. use of calcium channel blocking drugs, which may be associated with drug-induced-gingival-overgrowth).

8. *Hepato-biliary system* disorders or diseases may impact on the diagnosis or management of oral lesions. Normally the question asked relates to a history of jaundice or hepatitis. Other issues may include:
    *   Platelet levels and the risk of haemorrhage.
    *   Associated systemic diseases e.g. primary biliary cirrhosis (PBC) is associated with secondary Sjögren's syndrome.
    *   Drug metabolism may also be affected (the cytochrome P450 enzyme system).

9. *Gastro-intestinal tract* disease such as Crohn's, ulcerative colitis or coeliac disease may frequently present with oral manifestations. Malabsorption syndromes may lead to anaemia manifesting as oral ulceration or atrophic glossitis.

10. *Skin/dermatological disease* commonly presents with gingival manifestations, including erosive lichen planus, mucous membrane pemphigoid, pemphigus, Papillon Lèfevre Syndrome (PLS).

11. *Connective tissue diseases*, such as systemic sclerosis (scleroderma) or systemic lupus erythematosis (SLE) may have oral manifestations or require

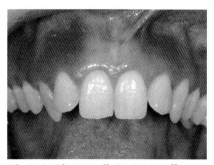 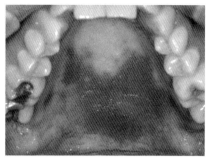

Fig 1-1a Plasma cell gingivitits affecting the gingivae and adjacent oral mucosa in a school telephonist who, when patch-tested, demonstrated sensitivity to a component of cleaning fluids used on the telephone mouthpiece.

Fig 1-1b The same condition as Fig 1-1a, affecting the hard palate. Similar lesions were evident in the larynx and the patient temporarily lost her voice. Both sets of lesions responded to systemic prednisolone therapy, prior to definitive diagnosis and implementation of preventive strategies.

    special precautions (e.g. 26% prevalence of cardiac valve damage is reported in SLE patients).

12. *Medications* must be comprehensively recorded, as many cause oral mucosal as well as periodontal lesions, such as lichenoid drug reactions, oral pigmentation, xerostomia, gingival overgrowth or ulcerative conditions.

13. *Allergies* may manifest within the gingivae and these may include coeliac disease, plasma cell gingivitis/mucositis (Fig 1-1).

14. *Immunodeficiency* should be recorded whether primary or secondary in nature, because this may affect subsequent management.

15. *Prion disease* should also be documented.

It is very helpful to include 'catch all' questions in the medical history questionnaire such as: 'Are you under any active treatment with your doctor?' or 'Have you ever been investigated in or admitted to hospital?' or 'Is there anything in your medical history we have not covered?'

As with the history of the complaint, it is often necessary to return to specific aspects of the medical history following the clinical examination.

Social History

Many aspects of a patient's social history may be of relevance to their presenting complaint.

<u>Specifically:</u>

Smoking - Are they a current or former smoker or someone who has never smoked (Box 1-1)?

Recreational drug use - Patients rarely volunteer the information that they are recreational drug users, but this may be relevant to their presenting pathology. Use of drugs such as amphetamines, cannabis, ecstasy or cocaine should be recorded and the method of use of cocaine may be particularly relevant (patients may rub it into their gingiva).

Alcohol consumption - Record the number of units taken per week and frequency of intake.

Diet - Diet can be particularly relevant to gingival and mucosal disease. This may involve recording fruit and vegetable intake, intake of erosive foods or those associated with allergy (e.g. cinnamaldehyde, benzoates).

Stress - Stress may be associated with conditions such as lichen planus and recurrent oral ulceration. Appropriate and sensitive questioning as to lifestyle and life events may be helpful.

Box 1-1 **Smoking History**

Current smoker	*Former smoker*	*Never smoked*
What do you smoke?	How many years did you smoke?	Are you exposed to passive smoking?
How many do you smoke?	How many per day?	At home or work?
For how many years?	What did you smoke?	How long for each day?
How soon after waking do you have your 1st cigarette?	When did you stop?	
Have you tried quitting?		
What went wrong?		

It is helpful to determine the patient's occupation at an early stage during the consultation. This may provide pointers towards causes of stress or indeed to other occupational hazards that may be contributing to the presenting complaint.

Habits – Habits may be the cause of traumatic oral lesions that can present with alarming signs and may also be associated with peripheral lesions.

Family History
The family history may be important for a number of reasons:
- It may help with establishing a diagnosis.
- It may provide indicators about prognosis and the natural history of the disease.

Sexual History
This is important in those cases where a sexually transmitted infection or HIV disease is considered a possibility. An explanation to the patient as to why you need such information is mandatory.

The extra-oral examination
The extra-oral examination should begin as soon as the patient enters the surgery. Dental surgeons must limit their examination to that of the clothed patient (Fig 1-2) and this does mean that their ability to arrive at a diagnosis may involve access to fewer pieces of evidence than their medical colleagues. Specifically note the patient's:
- Complexion – e.g. pallor/cyanosis/florid.
- Weight – may be relevant to increased risk of type 2 diabetes or other medical problems.
- Demeanour – does the patient look anxious, worried, embarrassed?
- Mobility – is this restricted physically or physiologically (case in Figs 5-5, 5-6 and 5-7).
- Skin condition – e.g. skin rashes.
- Facial appearance (Fig 1-3) – do not miss obvious facial indicators of systemic disease, e.g. SLE (rash).
- Verbal responses to questions – can reveal much about a patient's personality or fears.
- Exposed areas – examination of the clothed patient should also result in observation of hands, feet, scalp (Fig 1-4), neck, as well as facial features. Osteo- and rheumatoid arthritis, finger clubbing, nail pitting/dystrophy are all important clinical signs.

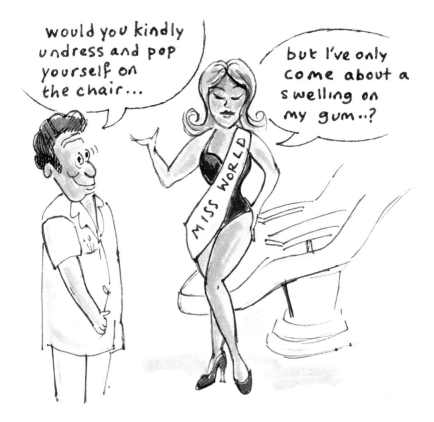

Fig 1-2 Dental surgeons must limit their examination to that of a clothed patient.

- Unexposed areas – sometimes it is necessary to view parts of a patient's skin that may be covered by clothing. This can be a sensitive matter and clinicians should use their discretion and ensure that a chaperone is present if appropriate. For example, lichen planus can present with itchy, purple papules on the flexor surfaces of the wrists or on the legs (Fig 1-5), which can help to determine a presumptive diagnosis.
- Lymphadenopathy – examination of the submandibular and submental regions along with the cervical chain of lymph nodes is vital when suspicious of infection or malignancy (Fig 1-6).
- Temporo-mandibular joints (TMJ) – TMJ examination may reveal clinical signs of joint pathology, parafunction or myofacial pain.

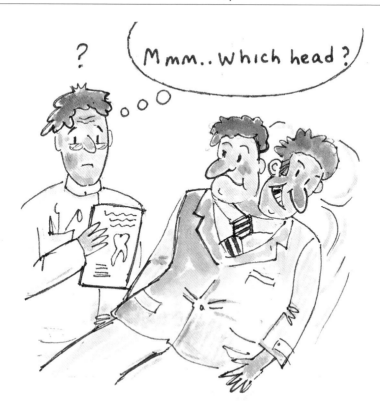

Fig 1-3 It is important not to miss obvious facial indicators of systemic disease.

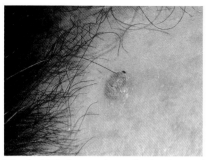

Fig 1-4 Viral wart along the hairline of the scalp of a male with gingival viral warts.

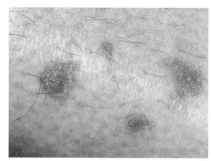

Fig 1-5 Purple 'pruritic' lesions, classical of lichen planus affecting the skin over the fibula and tibia of a 60-year-old female with erosive gingival lichen planus.

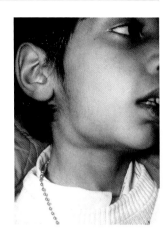

Fig 1-6 Right sub-mandibular lymphadenopathy in a five-year-old boy with oral Herpes simplex I infection.

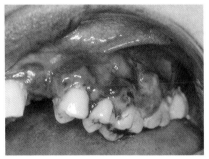

Fig 1-7 Triple pathology: lichen planus, NUG and pyostomatitis.

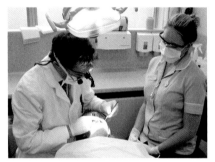

Fig 1-8 The use of loupes with fibre optic illumination.

The intra-oral examination
The intra-oral examination should follow a strict protocol or regime, to ensure no areas of the mouth or oropharynx are overlooked.

Examine the remainder of the mouth first, before the presenting lesions to ensure nothing else is missed that may be relevant to the diagnosis. Never assume the pathology is singular, dual and triple pathology may be evident (Fig 1-7).

Specifically ensure the following are examined systematically using good lighting and if necessary using magnification (Fig 1-8):
• Lips.
• Sulci.

- Cheeks (buccal mucosa parotid ducts, muscle attachments etc).
- Saliva flow from major ducts may be examined by massaging the gland and observing the colour and consistency of the saliva emerging from the relevant duct.
- Floor of mouth.
- Tongue – dorsum, anterior two-thirds, posterior third, lateral margins and ventral surface.
- Palate – hard and soft palate.
- Tonsillar region and oropharynx.
- Retro-molar regions.
- Gingivae.
- Teeth.

The floor of mouth and ventral surface of tongue shoulde be examined especially carefully as they are sites of sinister pathology.

When examining a lesion always supplement visual examination, by palpation, particularly the surface of the lesion. Be aware of any odour, e.g. foetor oris and if necessary use transillumination or bi-manual palpation. The latter, referred to as 'balloting' can be used for examining the submandibular salivary glands – one finger is placed in the lingual sulcus and one extraorally to roll the gland between, enabling assessment of fixity, consistency and size.

The Lesion
The following observations might be considered when examining lesions:
- Location?
- Nature of associated tissues?
- Size of the lesion?
- Shape of the lesion?
- Attachment to underlying structures?
- Colour?
- Surface characteristics?
- Nature of the base of the lesion?
- Consistency?
- Is there any associated pathology, locally or elsewhere on the body?
- Localised or generalised?

Location
The location of the lesion also gives a clue as to its origin and it is important to determine whether it remains localised to the free or attached gingivae or

extends beyond the mucogingival junction. In the latter case, a systemic condition is more likely (Fig 6-22).

When attempting to determine the origin of the lesion, consider the nature of those tissues that are present at the location, e.g. epithelial, vascular, neural, fibrous, fatty, glandular, bone, muscle.

Lesion size
When assessing the size of a lesion, one should also take into account its rate of growth, which may sometimes be determined from the patient's history. The lesion may be too large to excise without significant peri-operative morbidity and may require reconstructive surgery due to its size or the involvement of other tissue planes.

Lesion shape
The shape of a lesion may be very suggestive of its diagnosis. Care should be taken to examine the margins in particular. For example, an 'hour-glass shape' for an interdental swelling is indicative of a vascular epulis, and generalised shallow ulceration with ragged margins is characteristic, but not diagnostic of, mucosal herpes simplex (Fig 1-9).

Attachment
The nature of attachment of a lesion to the underlying tissues provides important diagnostic and prognostic information. A sessile lesion has a broad base and is therefore less likely to be a true epulis, since the latter are often pedunculated (borne on a pedicle). It is also important to determine whether the superficial tissues are fixed to underlying tissues or not, since this may indicate an invasive lesion.

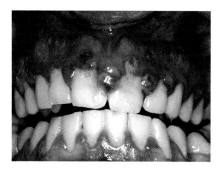

Fig 1-9 Gingival herpes simplex I infection.

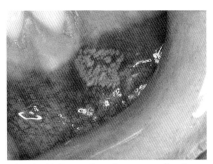

Fig 1-10 Ectopic sebaceous glands or 'Fordyce spots' located across the mucogingival junction in the LL34 area.

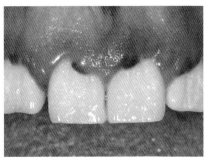

Fig 1-11 Pigmentation of gingival margins in an Afro-Caribbean woman, secondary to medication with zidovudine (AZT) for HIV-disease.

Colour

Red lesions may be inflammatory or vascular, whereas paler lesions may have a fibrous core. A yellow appearance may signify pus or fatty tissue. Fig 1-10 illustrates a common variation in normal anatomy at an unusual site, so-called 'Fordyce spots', which are ectopic sebaceous glands. Purple lesions indicate vascularity and brown or grey lesions are associated with melanin or other forms of pigmentation (e.g. amalgam debris, or drug-induced pigmentation – Fig 1-11 and 1-12).

Surface

The surface of a lesion provides important information about its nature. For example, an ulcerated surface may indicate trauma from opposing teeth, or necrosis due to an infection, trauma (e.g. acid burn - Fig 1-13) or indeed neoplasia. Surface keratosis may also indicate chronic trauma or true keratosis arising de-novo (Fig 1-14). It is also important to determine whether the surface can be removed or is adherent; a pseudomembrane would be typical of pseudomembranous candidosis.

Base

The base of a lesion may be helpful in provisional diagnosis. The granularity of an ulcer base suggests potentially sinister pathology.

Consistency

It is important always to 'feel' a lesion to determine its consistency or content. Mucosal and gingival lesions should be soft to touch, hard lesions

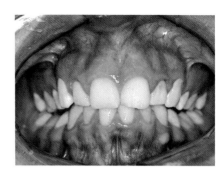

Fig 1-12 Purple pigmentation of the gingivae due to medication with the antibiotic minocycline for adolescent acne.

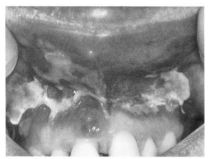

Fig 1-13 Surface necrosis of mucosal tissue following the misguided local application of aspirin for pain relief.

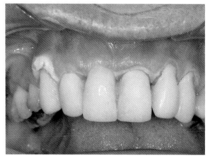

Fig 1-14 Linear gingival leukoplakia in a 50-year-old female who had never smoked and was a non-drinker. The tissue showed mild dysplasia histologically and an absence of candidal infection.

(induration) may be sinister or simply indicate underlying bone. Fluctuant lesions contain fluid, which may be pus or cyst fluid, and firm lesions may contain fibrous tissue.

Associated pathology
A vital part of the examination involves recognition of when an oral lesion may be related to disease elsewhere in the body. Such associated pathology may be visible as a sign (Fig 1-5) or may take the form of a symptom the patient may have withheld due to a perceived irrelevance to their gingival condition. For example, the six-year-old girl shown in Fig 1-15 had kidney pains and recurrent cystitis. Her kidney and liver function was mildly abnormal. However, consideration of the desquamative gingivitis, alongside abnormal renal and hepatic function, necessitated investigation for systemic lupus erythematosis (SLE), by serological methods (Chapter 2). Other con-

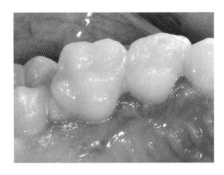

Fig 1-15 Desquamative gingivitis presenting in a six-year-old girl. Lichen planus has been described in children, but is extremely rare. Other potential diagnoses in this case included SLE.

ditions, such as Sjögrens syndrome, can be associated with primary biliary cirrhosis (PBC), and lichen planus can be associated with chronic active hepatitis, albeit rarely.

Localisation
Diagnostic clues can be derived from the distribution of the lesion(s). For example, solid tumours are more likely to be single as opposed to multiple (it is, however, acknowledged that approximately 20% of cases of oral squamous cell carcinoma may demonstrate multiple primaries). A bilateral lesion situated over major blood vessels may imply metastatic spread of a tumour (Fig 3-3). More widespread lesions tend to be associated with a systemic problem, for example drug-induced (Fig 6-9), hereditary (Fig 6-1), infective, immunological (Fig 1-1) or inflammatory (Figs 5-5 and 6-20) in nature.

The 'surgical sieve'
When attempting to formulate a differential diagnosis prior to performing special investigations, there may be occasions when the only thought entering the mind is 'I haven't got a clue' (Fig 1-16). Under these circumstances there are two options:
• Apply a surgical sieve.
• Refer the patient, providing as much information about the condition/lesion as possible (see above).

The surgical sieve comprises a series of headings, committed to memory, and which help to spark ideas and thoughts from generic principles. A mnemonic may be used to help memorise the sieve (Box 1-2).

Special Investigations
This subject will be covered in Chapter 2.

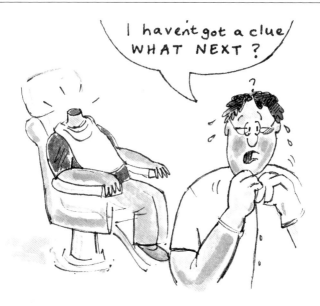

Fig 1-16 The 'Surgical Sieve'

Box 1-2

Heading	Mnemonic	Example
Metabolic/endocrine	M	Addisons disease (gingival pigmentation)
Inflammatory	I	Gingival angioedema (immunological)
Neoplastic	N	Gingival carcinoma
Infective	I	Gingival candidosis
Drug-induced	D	Gingival overgrowth or pigmentation
Hereditary	(H)	Hereditary gingival fibromatosis
Immunological	I	Plasma cell gingivitis
Not otherwise specified	N	
Trauma	T	Thermal, chemical or physical causes of ulceration

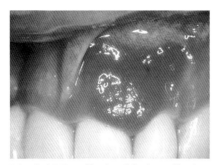

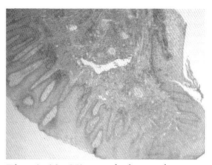

Fig 1-17 Localised red lesion affecting gingivae, but extending beyond mucogingival junction.

Fig 1-18 Histopathology shows a benign vascular lesion characteristic of a pyogenic granuloma.

The Differential Diagnosis

The objective of arriving at a 'differential diagnosis' is threefold:

- It informs the types of special clinical investigations required.
- It provides clinical details for the pathologist (or haematologist) of the most likely clinical diagnoses.
- It enables initial therapeutic strategies to be formulated. These may also serve a diagnostic function - for example, a swelling that responds to antimicrobial therapy, is most likely to be infective in origin.

Rarely, histological investigations may not help to determine a definitive diagnosis. The clinician may frequently be faced with a pathology report that requires careful interpretation alongside the historical and clinical information gathered. This approach is, in the author's opinion, the correct one, as exemplified by the case in Fig 1-17. In this case a vascular tumour was suspected clinically, but the histopathology was consistent with a benign pyogenic granuloma (Fig 1-18). The lesion spread and developed apparent satellite lesions within one week of the first biopsy (Fig 1-19) and a re-biopsy was performed. At review, the histopathology was still that of a benign vascular lesion, but the tumour was becoming exophytic (Fig 1-20). The urgency of the situation forced the clinician to re-explore a previously negative sexual history, and to ensure that the patient was clear that a diagnosis of Kaposi's sarcoma and therefore clinical AIDS was suspected. The patient subsequently revealed that he was homosexual and had practised unsafe sex. Counselling and a HIV serology test were immediately performed and HIV infection confirmed. On the basis of the historical and clinical information available, but contrary to the histopathological diagnosis, radiotherapy was performed and the lesion resolved (Fig 1-21).

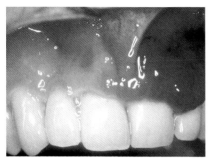

Fig 1-19 The lesion in Fig-1-17 one week post-primary incisional biopsy.

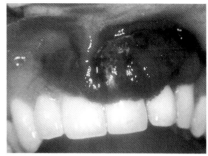

Fig 1-20 The lesion in Fig 1-17, 1 week after the second biopsy. The lesion has become exophytic and is spreading rapidly. The colour change reflects underlying areas of thrombosis and necrosis and blood congestion.

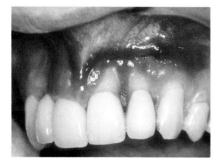

Fig 1-21 The treated lesion from 1-17 following external beam radiotherapy (in 1990) and residual pigmentation.

The Working Diagnosis

A presumptive (clinical) diagnosis is often sufficient for common lesions to enable the safe implementation of a therapeutic strategy. For example, desquamative gingivitis, where there is clear evidence of mucosal lichen planus (Fig 1-22), may be a presumptive clinical diagnosis for two reasons:

• Gingival biopsies are often of no diagnostic value for conditions such as lichen planus, because the inevitable presence of inflammation within the connective tissues, due to plaque accumulation, masks the more subtle features of lichen planus. Where possible, non-gingival biopsies should be employed (Fig 1-23).

• The clinical diagnosis may be so obvious (Fig 1-22) that it may not be appropriate to expose the patient to further investigations.

A further example would be pseudomembranous candidosis (Fig 1-24), where the implementation of topical antifungal therapy may resolve the condition before cytological results become available.

23

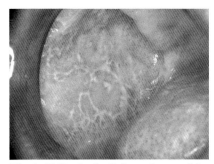

Fig 1-22 Reticular lichen planus of the left buccal mucosa is often a presumptive diagnosis. This should not be the case for erosive lichen planus, where a small but nevertheless increased risk of malignant transformation exists.

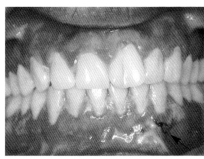

Fig 1-23 A biopsy has been taken below the muco-gingival line, to avoid plaque-induced gingival inflammation masking features of lichen planus.

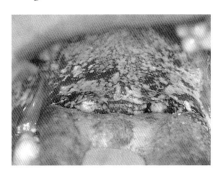

Fig 1-24 Florid pseudomembranous candidosis (thrush) of the palate in an HIV-positive patient.

Definitive Diagnosis

A definitive diagnosis is one in which the diagnosis is as certain as possible based on a thorough history, examination and investigation. Such a diagnosis forms the basis of treatment strategies, but it is vital to remember that diagnoses can change during the course of a disease. For example, a patient initially managed for localised aggressive periodontitis (LAP), may in later life develop a chronic periodontitis due to local risk factors encouraging plaque accumulation (e.g. interproximal recession due to former LAP). Squamous cell carcinoma may develop within erosive lichen planus.

Also bear in mind that multiple pathology may be concurrent in the same patient and therefore always keep an open mind as to differential, presumptive and working diagnoses. The patient illustrated in Fig 1-7 has triple pathology at presentation:

- NUG.
- Erosive lichen planus.
- Pyostomatitis vegetans.

Key Points

- Approach each case with an open mind and be prepared for changes in diagnosis or multiple pathology.
- Explore all aspects of the patient's complaint and its history in a forensic manner.
- Be aware of the need to follow certain branches of the medical history to their conclusion and recognise when to terminate other lines of questioning.
- Always return to the history in the light of new information and be prepared to re-appraise matters.
- Remember to collect family, social and lifestyle histories, including habits, diet, tobacco and alcohol consumption, stress and coping behaviours for stress.
- Examine all visible areas of the clothed patient and do not miss the obvious.
- Use a systematic and thorough approach to the intra-oral examination with good lighting and magnification.
- Use all senses and don't just rely upon what you can see.
- Record your findings carefully and logically.
- Examine associated pathology.
- Use of the surgical sieve can be a helpful approach.
- Always seek a second opinion whenever in doubt.

Further Reading

Chapple ILC, Gilbert AD (eds). Understanding Periodontal Diseases: Assessment and Diagnostic Procedures in Practice. London: Quintessentials, 2002:67.

Chapter 2
The Role of Clinical Investigations

Aim

The aim of this chapter is to allude to those clinical investigations that are of value in formulating a definitive diagnosis.

Outcome

Having understood this chapter, the reader should be aware of those relevant investigations that are used to either confirm diagnoses or add information to help formulate a definitive diagnosis. The reader will be aware of the need to identify appropriate investigations for particular conditions and, in addition, understand the limitations and interpretation of those investigations.

Introduction

The number of investigative procedures now available is extensive and continues to expand with advances in technology. It should be borne in mind that while investigations are a most important step in the clinical management of many patients, they must not be used as a substitute for a detailed clinical history and examination.

General Considerations

Before embarking upon any investigative procedure, a variety of general factors need to be considered. These include the nature and safety of the test, its potential benefit to the patient, any possible adverse effects, its cost effectiveness and whether the result is likely to alter the management of the patient's condition. Undertaking investigative procedures for the sake of interest is unacceptable. The patient must be fully informed of the need for the investigation, its advantages and disadvantages, including possible adverse events, before proceeding. As in all aspects of patient care, the balance of risk of an investigation must favour the patient.

When requesting investigative procedures, the following considerations should be borne in mind:
• What information is required?
• Which test(s) will provide that information?
• How are the results interpreted?

Indications for Investigation

Whilst investigative procedures are predominantly used to support or confirm a clinical suspicion or diagnosis, they may also be used to:
• exclude abnormalities.
• monitor disease activity/progression.
• measure response to therapy.

Interpretation of Investigations

The results of any investigation must be interpreted with caution so as to avoid drawing erroneous conclusions that may lead to inappropriate patient management. For example, in serological investigations:

• Slightly abnormal results should be repeated for confirmation. They may be within the methodological variance for the assay.
• Compare results with previous values (if available) to ascertain any trend or change.
• Compare results with other associated parameters to ascertain consistency.
• Identify possible artefacts.

The normal range is usually taken as the mean ± 2 standard deviations, i.e. 95% of the population fall within that range. It is therefore important to recognise that results outside the normal range may be 'normal' for a particular patient and may not signal anything untoward, especially if the result is not corroborated by other test results.

Specificity and Sensitivity of Tests

It is important when interpreting investigations to have some understanding of the specificity and sensitivity of the investigations concerned. An important area for such considerations is when testing for autoantibodies. For example, the finding of certain autoantibodies does not necessarily confirm the presence of a particular disease, whilst equally, their absence may not preclude that disease.

The specificity of a test is defined as:
- The percentage of people without the disease who have a negative test result, e.g. 95% specificity implies 5% false positive results.

The sensitivity of a test is defined as:
- The percentage of people with the disease who have a positive test result, e.g. 95% sensitivity implies 5% false negative results.

Biopsy

Tissue biopsy and subsequent histological examination remains a particularly valuable investigation in the diagnosis of gingival and oral mucosal disease. Although the technique is usually straightforward, it is essential to ensure that the pathologist receives a diagnostic sample that is not compromised, either by injection of local anaesthetic solution directly into the biopsy specimen, or traumatic handling of the tissue either at the time of the surgery or subsequently.

As with all clinical investigations, the request form that will accompany the specimen must be accurately and fully completed, providing details of the clinical features of the condition, the patient's medical history, including details of any medication and a differential diagnosis.

When undertaking gingival biopsies, it is important to consider that histological interpretation can be confounded due to the level of background inflammatory change that is usually present within the gingival tissues. For this reason, it may be preferable to biopsy alternative sites if appropriate (Fig 2-1).

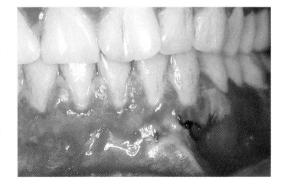

Fig 2-1 Slide demonstrating a suture placed at a para-gingival biopsy site. A gingival biopsy has been avoided to provide a representative sample devoid of the chronic inflammation often found within gingival biopsies secondary to plaque accumulation.

The following considerations will help ensure that a diagnostic biopsy sample is obtained:

- Avoid injecting local anaesthetic directly into the tissue to be removed.
- Do not tear or crush the tissue during the procedure.
- Excise a representative sample of the lesion.
- Additionally, excise any areas that differ from the overall appearance of the lesion. This may necessitate multiple sampling.
- Remove an adequate size of tissue. Aim for approximately 8-10mm in diameter and ensure that subepithelial tissues are included.
- Avoid biopsying an ulcer alone – by definition there will be no epithelium and this will compromise histological diagnosis.
- Perilesional tissue is often of diagnostic value.
- Place the specimen on a piece of card (e.g. the suture card) or paper, cut-side down, to reduce curling of the specimen and shrinkage.
- Ensure that the specimen is put into an appropriate volume of fixative if routine histological examination is required.
- Ensure the specimen is not put into fixative if special staining techniques such as direct immunofluorescence are to be employed. Fresh tissue should be transported to the laboratory in saline-soaked gauze or appropriate transport media such as 'Michel's' medium. Direct immunofluorescence may be particularly useful when autoimmune vesiculobullous disease is suspected (Fig 2-2).

The histological findings do not always support the clinical diagnosis and in some cases, ultimately a judgement must be made as to the definitive diagnosis. A high index of suspicion is always advisable, particularly in those circumstances where sinister pathology is suspected clinically, but not supported histologically. Reappraisal of the original biopsy specimen with consideration of a further biopsy or biopsies is appropriate in such cases.

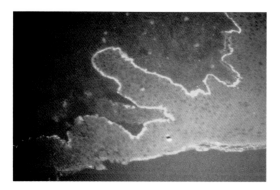

Fig 2-2 Direct immunofluorescence staining of mucous membrane pemphigoid showing IgG deposition at the basement membrane.

Microbiology

When infection is suspected, various investigations may be helpful to identify the aetiological agent.

Identification of Bacteria

Culture of organisms from oral swabs is frequently undertaken and combined with antibiotic sensitivity testing. However, results can be difficult to interpret because of the background level of oral commensal organisms. The initially sterile swab should be moistened in sterile normal saline or water to enhance the harvest and then passed over the area of interest before being placed back in its sterile container and sent to the laboratory without delay. If the patient is already taking antibiotics, this will confound the results.

Culture of specific periodontal bacteria requires the use of dedicated transport and culture media for fastidious organisms, together with the appropriate laboratory expertise, and is rarely indicated. Recombinant DNA probe technology overcomes these issues but as selection of antimicrobial regimes remains somewhat broad, rather than being highly targeted at specific species, there are few indications for such investigations in routine clinical practice.

Other tests, such as identification of specific serum antibodies, can also be undertaken. Rapid immunological assays to identify either specific antigens or antibodies are also available, but not commonly indicated for most gingival pathologies.

Gingival smears can also be used to identify specific organisms under the light microscope.

Identification of Fungal Organisms

For identification of the presence of fungal organisms, such as Candida species, swabs can also be used. They require to be cultured on the appropriate selective growth medium (Sabouraud's agar), but since commensal carriage of these organisms is common (50% of individuals), a positive culture per se does not necessarily indicate active infection. Semi-quantitative methods such as imprint cultures and oral rinses can also be used, provided the receiving laboratory has the necessary equipment to perform the test. A simpler alternative is the smear, where a flat plastic instrument is used to gently scrape the surface mucosa, the material so removed being smeared on a glass slide and fixed. Subsequent staining with PAS or Gram stains and examination under the light microscope will show the fungal

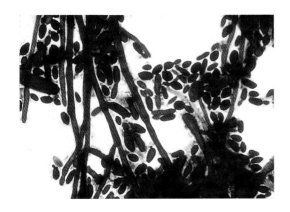

Fig 2-3 PAS-stained smear demonstrating hyphal and yeast forms of Candida albicans.

organisms (Fig 2-3). The presence of the mycelial form of the organism is suggestive of clinical infection rather than commensal carriage.

Speciation of organisms can also be undertaken, using commercial kits that may differentiate species on the basis of germ tube production or fermentation of sugars.

Identification of Viruses
The presence of a virus can be confirmed by various techniques, including that of culture. However, obtaining a viral culture is a more complex process than that for bacteria and fungal organisms, as it requires the provision of live cells as opposed to simple growth media.

Tissue biopsy or cytology may be helpful as the presence of cytopathic effects (e.g. Mulberry nuclei) indicates the presence of viral pathology, although not necessarily a specific virus type (Fig 2-4). Additionally, harvesting vesicle fluid and subsequent electron microscopy can be used to identify virions.

Serological testing for specific acute and convalescent antibody titres can be used to demonstrate viral infection, with a four-fold rise in antibody titre being taken as a positive result. However, as the result becomes available once the patient has recovered, such testing is of limited practical value in managing the patient. Newer, rapid techniques that identify specific viral antigens or antibodies, based on immunofluorescence or enzyme linked immunosorbent assays (ELISA) are now available which abrogate the requirement for paired samples.

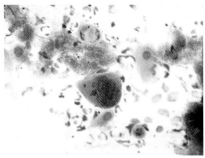

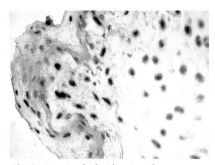

Fig 2-4 Smear demonstrating cytopathic effect in Herpes simplex infection (Tzanck cells and ballooning degeneration).

Fig 2-5 In situ hybridisation demonstrating the presence of Epstein Barr virus.

Molecular biology techniques also allow rapid identification of viral nucleic acid, for example, the polymerase chain reaction or in situ hybridisation. Both techniques provide rapid highly specific results but require specialised equipment (Fig 2-5).

It is essential to discuss the case with the virology laboratory to ensure that the most suitable test is requested and that the appropriate sample is sent to the laboratory.

Blood and Serological Tests

A large range of tests is available. Laboratories will often group tests together to allow broad screening for a variety of disease entities. This can encourage some clinicians to effectively undertake a 'fishing exercise' looking for a range of serological parameters, as opposed to being specific in their requests. This is not good clinical practice, being wasteful of resource and is usually unhelpful. As always, investigations must be regarded as an adjunct to undertaking a careful history and examination and not a replacement for these skills.

When requesting blood or serological investigations, the specimen must be collected in the appropriate container for the required test. If there is uncertainty as to the nature of the blood collection tube required, advice should be sought from the laboratory. Additionally, some specimens require to be mixed with an anticoagulant contained within the blood collection tube. Failure to do this will result in a sample that cannot be used for the assay. Prolonged venous stasis should be avoided during venepuncture, as this can introduce inaccuracies in the measurement of certain components, especially those that are bound to plasma proteins such as calcium.

Table 2-1 and Table 2-2 provide a brief summary of some of the more frequently requested blood and serological investigations used in specialist practice.

Identification of autoantibodies does not necessarily indicate the presence of the disease that is usually associated with that autoantibody. Conversely, lack of circulating antibodies does not preclude the diagnosis of the associated disease.

Considerations such as specificity and sensitivity of the test, age and gender of the patient and titre of the antibody are important in test interpretation. The finding of weak positives, as for any test, must be interpreted with great caution and corroborative evidence can be helpful in this regard.

It is most important that the patient is not stigmatised as a consequence of inappropriate interpretation of the results of clinical investigations.

Radiology and Imaging

This subject is beyond the scope of this text and is comprehensively covered in Panoramic Radiology and 21st Century Dental Imaging of this series. Additionally, Chapter 11 addresses periodontal conditions with radiological features.

Further Reading

Horner K (ed). Panoramic Radiology. London: Quintessentials, 2005.

Horner K (ed), Twenty-first Century Dental Imaging. London: Quintessentials, 2005.

Marshall WJ, Baugert SK. Clinical Chemistry. 5th edition. London: Mosby, 2004.

McGhee M. A Guide To Laboratory Investigation. 4th edition. Oxford: Radcliffe Medical Press, 2003.

Table 2-1 **Blood investigations commonly used in periodontal medicine**

Investigation	Indication	Comments
Full blood count	Anaemias/ myeloproliferative or myelosuppressive disease	
Serum ferritin	Iron deficiency anaemia/ iron overload	Ferritin also behaves as an acute phase marker – elevated levels do not necessarily indicate iron overload
Serum folate	Oral ulceration, candidosis, stomatitis Red cell macrocytosis ± anaemia apparant from full blood count	Serum folate levels are labile. Red cell folate is a more stable measure but more costly to perform. Never give folate supplementation to patients with low serum B12 levels. This will cause remaining B12 stores to be metabolised, resulting in possible neurological complications
Serum B12	Oral ulceration, candidosis, stomatitis. Red cell macrocytosis ± anaemia /pancytopaenia apparent from full blood count	Low B12 is rarely due to dietary deficiency. Consider other causes such as pernicious anaemia, ileal disease or partial gastrectomy

Investigation	Indication	Comments
Blood glucose	Oral candidosis Multiple periodontal abscesses	If random blood glucose abnormal, consider fasting glucose level
Clinical chemistry (including liver function tests)	Suspected metabolic bone disease, electrolyte disturbance, liver, renal & endocrine, disease e.g. alkaline phosphatase for hypophosphatasia	
Liver function tests		
Erythrocyte sedimentation rate	Of little diagnostic value in most circumstances	Very non-specific index of inflammation. More useful in tracking disease activity and response to therapy. ESR is helpful in supporting a diagnosis of temporal arteritis
C reactive protein	As for ESR	

Table 2-2 **Autoantibody investigations commonly used in periodontal medicine**

Autoantibody Tests	Disease Association	Comments
Anti-nuclear antibodies	Systemic lupus erythematosus (SLE)	May also be found in other connective tissue diseases but not in discoid lupus erythematosus (anti-double strand DNA antibodies are diagnostic of active SLE and high titres carry a poor prognosis.)
Rheumatoid factor	Seropositive rheumatoid arthritis	May be found in other connective tissue diseases
Antibodies to extractable nuclear antigens (ENA)	Sjogren's syndrome (Anti-Ro, & /or Anti-La) Systemic sclerosis (ScL70) SLE (anti-Ro, anti-Sm)	A family of antibodies to non-nucleoprotein soluble nuclear antigens producing a speckled pattern of immunofluorescence.
ANCA–C (Cytoplasmic staining)	Wegener's granulomatosis	ANCA–C (anti-proteinase 3) has a high specificity for Wegener's granulomatosis.
ANCA-P (Perinuclear staining)	Granulomatous conditions such as Crohn's disease	ANCA–P targets myeloperoxidase
Anti-gastric parietal cell	Pernicious anaemia	High sensitivity but low specificity
Anti-intrinsic factor	Pernicious anaemia	High specificity

Autoantibody Tests	Disease Association	Comments
Anti-basement membrane zone	Pemphigoid	
Anti-intercellular cement	Pemphigus	Anti-desmoglein 3 antibodies are found in mucosal and cutaneous pemphigus. Anti-desmoglein 1 occurs predominantly in cutaneous pemphigus
Anti-endomysial Anti-tissue transglutaminase	Coeliac disease Coeliac disease	These are much more sensitive and specific markers for coeliac disease and have largely replaced anti-reticulin and IgA isotype anti-gliadin antibodies

Chapter 3
Gingival Colour Changes – Localised

Aim

The aim of this chapter is to describe those gingival colour changes that are localised in one area or, in some cases, several discrete areas of the gingivae.

Outcome

Having read this chapter, the reader should have an increased awareness of the nature of local gingival colour changes, their clinical significance and appropriate management, including differential diagnosis and treatment if indicated. The contents of this chapter are summarised in Table 3-1.

Red Lesions

It is important to consider that some localised red lesions may represent periodontal sepsis, for example a lateral periodontal abscess, but this will be discussed in Chapter 5.

Kaposi's Sarcoma

Kaposi's sarcoma occurs in more than 50% of patients with AIDS, becoming increasingly frequent as the disease progresses. Oral involvement may be the initial site of presentation, and gingival involvement is common. This condition may present as an epulis, perhaps mimicking a vascular pyogenic granuloma.

Clinical appearance
- Clinical appearance is variable, light (Fig 3-1), dark red (Fig 3-2), purple/blue or even de-pigmented lesions having been described.
- Sessile macules/papules which may also have a nodular surface and become exophytic.
- Satellite lesions may develop.

Clinical symptoms
- Usually asymptomatic but patients may complain about the aesthetics or of bleeding following trauma.

Table 3–1 **Summary table – localised gingival colour changes**

Major Categories	Sub Categories	Frequency of Condition	Management Setting
Red lesions	Kaposi's sarcoma	Rare	Specialist referral for diagnostic confirmation and investigation of immune status
	Arteriovenous malformations/ haemangiomata	Uncommon	Many lesions require no active intervention other than reassurance
	Telangiectasia	Uncommon	No active intervention required but may need to investigate for underlying disease – best undertaken in specialist units
	Erythroplakia	Very rare	A sinister lesion. Urgent referral to secondary care for diagnosis and appropriate treatment
White lesions	Trauma	Common	Primary care
	Leukoplakia	Uncommon on the gingivae	Biopsy and monitoring can be undertaken in primary care. More extensive lesions should be managed in specialist units

Major Categories	Sub Categories	Frequency of Condition	Management Setting
	White sponge naevus	Rare	Diagnosis will usually be the remit of specialist units. No active treatment is required and there is no known malignant potential
	Squamous cell carcinoma	Very uncommon on the gingivae	Urgent referral to specialist units
	Lichen planus	Common	Recalcitrant lichen planus should be referred to specialist units for diagnostic confirmation, treatment and monitoring
	Candidosis	Gingival involvement is very rare	Referral to specialist units for further investigations
Pigmented lesions	Amalgam tattoo	Common	Primary care or referral if diagnosis is in doubt
	Melanotic macule	Uncommon	Primary care or referral if diagnosis is in doubt
	Naevi	Uncommon	Primary care or referral if diagnosis is in doubt
	Malignant melanoma	Very rare	Urgent referral to specialist unit

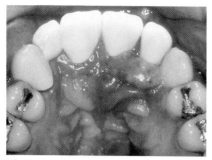

Fig 3-1 Kaposi's sarcoma that is pale in appearance.

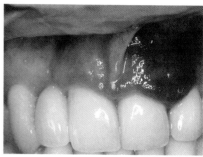

Fig 3-2 Kaposi's sarcoma that is dark red in appearance.

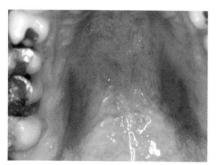

Fig 3-3 Kaposi's following the greater palatine neurovascular bundle.

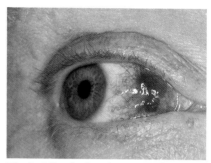

Fig 3-4 Ocular involvement of Kaposi's sarcoma.

Aetiology
- Human herpes virus 8 (HHV8) – a gamma herpes virus is strongly associated with the aetiology of KS.

Involvement of non-gingival sites
- The palate is the most common site of intra-oral involvement, particularly following the course of the greater palatine neurovascular bundles (Fig 3-3).
- Skin lesions.
- Ocular lesions (Fig 3-4).
- Visceral involvement.

Differential diagnosis
- Haemangiomata/Arterio-venous malformations.

- Inflammatory hyperplasias, e.g. pyogenic granuloma or peripheral giant cell lesions.
- Periodontal abscess.
- Localised plasma cell gingivitis.
- Localised lesions of Molluscum contageosum.
- Pigmented lesions including malignant melanoma.
- Bacillary angiomatosis (secondary to Bartonella henselae/quintana infection).

Clinical investigation
- Definitive diagnosis is by incisional biopsy, though lesions can appear benign and histologically identical to a pyogenic granuloma.
- Careful medical and sexual histories are crucial to aid presumptive diagnosis.
- In-situ polymerase chain reaction (PCR) may be used, where available, to identify HHV8 within the tumours.

Management options
- Lesions are often multifocal, and thus further medical examination is necessary to identify the distribution of all lesions.
- Highly active anti-retroviral therapy (HAART) may affect resolution of the lesions.
- Chemotherapy.
- In early lesions local management may be indicated, (e.g. intralesional vincristine, surgical excision).

Vascular Lesions
Clinical features
- Vascular lesions that affect the gingivae are an uncommon clinical finding.
- Colour varies from blue/red/purple.
- They may be flat or more commonly elevated.
- Usually asymptomatic.
- Blanching occurs on pressure as the vessels are emptied.
- Occasionally they may bleed, eg if traumatised.

Aetiology
- Haemangiomata - developmental lesions that are present from birth and spontaneously regress with age (Fig 3-5).
- Arterio-venous malformations (Fig 3-6).

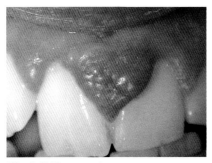

Fig 3-5 Haemangioma.

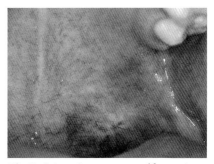

Fig 3-6 Arterio-venous malformation.

Involvement of non-gingival sites
- Tongue.
- Lip.
- Any area can be involved, intra-orally or extra-orally.

Differential diagnosis
- Telangiectasia.
- Purpura.
- Kaposi's sarcoma.
- Lymphangioma.

Clinical investigation
- Aspiration.
- Imaging to identify extent and distribution of the lesion (MRI, Doppler ultrasound).
- Angiography.

Management options
- Usually require no active treatment.
- Cryosurgery (Fig 3-7).
- Laser.
- Sclerosing solutions.
- Embolisation of feeder vasculature.

Telangiectasia
Telangiectasia, are capillary blood vessel dilatations and may occur peri-orally and intra-orally. They are uncommon on the gingival tissues (Fig 3-8).

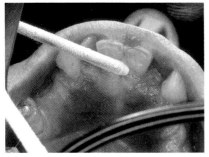

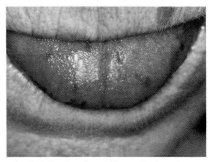

Fig 3-7 Cryosurgery to an arterio-venous malformation.

Fig 3-8 Perioral and lingual telangiectasia in a patient with limited systemic sclerosis.

Clinical appearance
• Small red macules, often multiple, which blanch on pressure.

Clinical symptoms
• Telangiectasia are usually asymptomatic but may bleed on trauma.

Aetiology
• Congenital or developmental depending on the type.

Involvement of non-gingival sites
• Telangiectasia may occur on any skin or mucosal surface as well as involving the viscera.

Differential diagnosis
• Hereditary haemorrhagic telangiectasia (Osler-Weber-Rendu syndrome)
  - Cutaneous and gastrointestinal tract involvement is common.
  - Epistaxis is also a frequent accompanying feature.
• Limited systemic sclerosis (previously known as 'CREST' syndrome – an acronym for: Calcinosis, Raynaud's phenomenon, Esophagitis, Sclerodactyly and Telangiectasia). See Chapter 10.

Clinical investigation
• The diagnosis is usually made on clinical history and examination.

Management options
• No active intervention is usually indicated.

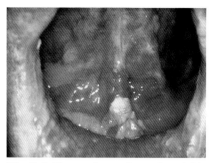 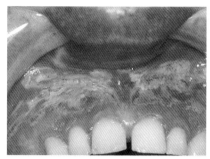

Fig 3-9 Floor of mouth erythroplakia with a squamous cell carcinoma centrally.

Fig 3-10 Aspirin burn of the gingival and alveolar mucosa.

Erythroplakia (Erythroplasia)
Clinical features (Reichart 2005)
- A rare lesion.
- Appears as an atrophic, flat velvety red patch. (Fig 3-9)
- Very high incidence of dysplasia or frank malignancy – erythroplakia should be regarded as malignant until histologically proven otherwise.
- More common in middle aged/elderly males.

Aetiology
- Unknown.

Involvement of non-gingival sites
- May occur at any oral mucosal site as well as at other mucosal sites.
- Most commonly, floor of mouth, ventral surface of the tongue and palate.

Differential diagnosis
- Inflammatory lesions (lichen planus, erythema migrans).
- Candidosis.

Clinical investigation
- Biopsy is mandatory to identify dysplastic or neoplastic changes, which are the usual findings.

Management options
- Excision with wide margin due to the high risk of malignant transformation.
- Avoidance of risk factors (tobacco and alcohol).

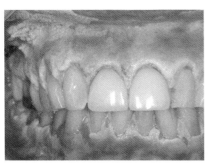

Fig 3-11 Leukoplakia of the gingiva.

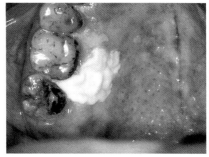

Fig 3-12 Dense leukoplakia of the hard palate and attached gingiva as a result of reverse smoking.

• Advice on a diet rich in anti-oxidants (empirical).
• Careful monitoring at short intervals.

White Lesions

Trauma
Chemical, physical or thermal trauma can produce red, white or ulcerated lesions on the gingiva and oral mucosa. Perhaps the best-known example is that of a local chemical burn arising as a consequence of dissolving an aspirin tablet on the gingiva adjacent to a painful tooth. The patient's history usually elicits the cause of the trauma and these lesions resolve spontaneously (Fig 3-10).

Leukoplakia
A leukoplakia is an adherent white patch that cannot be categorised as any other morphological or histological diagnosis.

Clinical features
• Gingiva is not a common site of involvement (Fig 3-11).
• Leukoplakias are premalignant lesions. Approximately 4% of lesions will transform to a squamous cell carcinoma over 10–20 years (Rhodus, 2005).
• Clinical risk features include:
  – Density (Fig 3-12).
  – Verrucous surface.
  – Floor of mouth/ventral tongue.
  – Erythema.
  – Ulceration.

- Hyperplastic margins.
- Sudden change in lesions.
- Spontaneous pain.

Aetiology
- Idiopathic.
- Habits.
  - Smoking.
  - Alcohol.
  - Betel nut chewing.
- Chronic Trauma (friction).
  Sharp teeth/teeth opposing edentulous ridge.
- Actinic radiation.
- Systemic disease (uncommon).
  - Plummer Vinson syndrome.
  - Renal dialysis.
  - Syphilis.

Involvement of non-gingival sites
- Leukoplakias may occur at any site, but the floor of the mouth and ventral surface of the tongue appear to be at increased risk of malignant transformation (20%) (Fig 3-13).

Differential diagnosis
- Candidosis.
- Lichen planus.
- Discoid lupus erythematosus.
- Skin grafts.
- Burns (chemical or thermal).
- Congenital (e.g. Leukokeratosis mucosae oris).

Clinical investigation
- Biopsy – the clinical appearance is often a poor guide to the histological features.
- Microbiology.
- Haematology if clinically indicated, although routinely this is inappropriate.

Management options
- Identify and eliminate contributory factors, e.g. smoking, alcohol, sharp teeth, candidal infection.

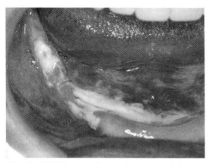

Fig 3-13 Floor of mouth leukoplakia.

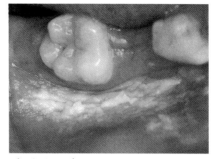

Fig 3-14 White sponge naevus involving the gingiva.

- Long term review or excise lesion - this is dependent on clinical features, patient's state of health and biopsy results (i.e. degree of dysplasia.)
- Advise patient to return immediately if they notice any sudden change in the character or behaviour of the lesion.
- Encourage diet rich in anti-oxidants (empirical advice).
- Possible value of toluidine blue staining in long term monitoring.
- Consider identification of human papillomavirus (type 16) in proliferative veruccous leukoplakias.

Leukokeratosis Mucosae Oris (White Sponge Naevus of Cannon)

Leukokeratosis mucosae oris is an uncommon developmental anomaly that in some patients may be extensive. The condition is not regarded as being premalignant.

Clinical features
- Asymptomatic localised or more generalised hyperkeratosis that is somewhat folded and often quite thickened (Fig 3-14).
- A large area or areas of mucosa may be involved.
- The condition usually presents in childhood.
- Gingival involvement is very uncommon.

Aetiology
- Autosomal dominant inheritance.
- Mutations in keratin genes for the mucosal-specific keratins, K4 and K13 (Rugg et al 1999).

Involvement of non-gingival sites
- Buccal mucosa.
- Ventral surface of the tongue/floor of the mouth.
- Alveolar mucosa.
- Labial mucosa.
- Palate.
- Extra-oral involvement may include nasal, genital and ano-rectal mucosa.

Differential diagnosis
- Pachyonychia congenita.
- Hereditary benign intraepithelial dysplasia (Witkop's disease).
- Mechanical trauma, e.g. cheek biting.
- Leukoedema.
- Leukoplakia.
- Pseudomembranous candidosis.

Clinical investigation
- Histological examination.

Management options
- No active treatment is required.
- Anecdotal reports exist that in some cases the condition may respond favourably to systemic antibiotics such as the tetracyclines.

Squamous Cell Carcinoma

Oral sqaumous cell carcinoma may present variously as white or red patches, warty, or granular lesions, swellings or ulcers. White patches that suddenly show clinical change, are densely white, speckled, warty or ulcerated are similarly suspicious and should be biopsied urgently. A fuller account of oral squamous cell carcinoma will be found in Chapter 7.

Lichen Planus

Oral lichen planus, or more typically oral lichenoid reactions, may unusually present as localised lesions as opposed to the condition's classical bilateral and often widespread distribution. This may be seen, for example, adjacent to amalgam restorations in susceptible patients. A full account of oral lichen planus may be found in Chapter 4.

Candidosis

Gingival candidosis is rare and when it occurs, other than when it is denture- associated, may indicate underlying immunosuppression. Whilst Can-

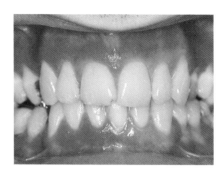

Fig 3-15 Gingival candidosis in a patient with HIV disease.

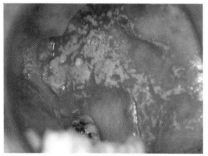

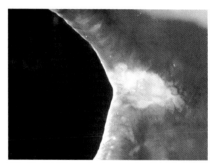

Fig 3-16 Acute pseudomembranous candidosis (thrush).

Fig 3-17 Chronic hyperplastic candidosis at the anterior commissure (candidal leukoplakia).

dida albicans is the most prevalent organism, other species such as C. tropicalis or C. glabrata may also be identified. It is also pertinent to note that gingival candidal infections may present as red rather than white areas of mucosa (Fig 3-15).

Clinical features
Candidosis may present intra-orally in a variety of different forms:
- Acute pseudomembraneous – white plaques that can be removed to leave an underlying erythematous surface (Fig 3-16).
- Acute atrophic – diffuse red appearance that may result from the use of broad spectrum antibiotics and inhaled corticosteroids.
- Chronic hyperplastic – typically a triangular, speckled lesion at the anterior commissures (Fig 3-17).
- Chronic mucocutaneous – widespread lesions often affecting the tongue and producing dystrophic nail changes, as well as affecting other mucocutaneous sites (Fig 3-18).

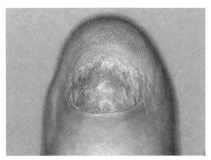

Fig 3-18 Dystrophic nail changes in chronic mucocutaneous candidosis.

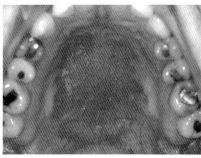

Fig 3-19 Chronic erythematous candidosis as a presenting sign of HIV disease.

- Chronic erythematous – diffuse erythema that mimics denture stomatitis and may be seen in HIV/AIDS infections (Fig 3-19).
- Candidosis is usually painless although the atrophic/erythematous variants may produce soreness.

Aetiology
- Local factors
  - Denture wearing.
  - Smoking.
  - Xerostomia.
  - Topical steroid therapy.

- Systemic factors
  - Diabetes mellitus.
  - Haematinic deficiency.
  - Medication (corticosteroids, broad spectrum antibiotics, chemotherapy).
  - Immunosuppressive states including HIV/AIDS.
  - Candidosis endocrinopathy syndrome (rare) – a variant of chronic mucocutaneous candidosis, where there is multiple endocrine pathology including autoimmune thyroid, parathyroid and adrenal hypofunction.

Involvement of non-gingival sites
- Any intra-oral site can be involved.
- Chronic hyperplastic candidosis typically affects the anterior commissural region.
- Acute atrophic candidosis usually involves the distal hard/soft palate.
- Chronic mucocutaneous candidosis also affects the skin and nail beds.

Differential diagnosis
- White or red lesions of the oral mucosa including:
  - Leukoplakia.
  - Lichen planus.
  - Erythroplakia.

Clinical investigation
- Swabs for culture (semi-quantitative methods such as imprint cultures or oral rinses are available in some laboratories).
- Smears for visual identification of hyphae which are indicative of active infection as opposed to commensal carriage.
- Biopsy in the case of suspected chronic hyperplastic candidosis – this condition is premalignant; 50% of cases demonstrate dysplastic change histologically. Although this may be reactive in some cases, 9–40% of lesions are reported to undergo malignant transformation.
- Full blood count.
- Haematinics.
- Blood glucose.

Management options
- Eliminate local factors.
- Eliminate/treat systemic factors.
- Anti-fungal agents.
- Long term review for chronic hyperplastic candidosis (malignant potential).

Pigmented Lesions

Amalgam Tattoo
Clinical features
- A flat, grey/blue discolouration of the mucosa, resulting from amalgam particles (or other metals) becoming impacted in the soft tissue which subsequently becomes stained as metal ions leach out into the tissues (Figs 3-20 and 3-21).
- One of the most common causes of a discrete area of intra-oral hyperpigmentation.
- They may gradually enlarge and darken with time.
- The lesion is asymptomatic.
- Frequently involves the gingivae.

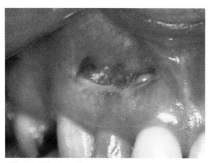

Fig 3-20 Amalgam tattoo.

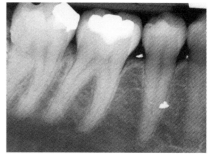

Fig 3-21 Radiograph showing underlying amalgam particles in the tissues of an amalgam tattoo.

Aetiology
- Amalgam becoming impacted into the soft tissues during restorative dental procedures.

Involvement of non-gingival sites
- Any mucosal site close to the teeth is potentially liable to trauma and subsequent impaction of foreign material into the soft tissue.
- Mucosal flaps raised in apicectomy wounds may show amalgam tattoos as a consequence of the use of amalgam as the retrograde filling material.

Differential diagnosis
- Racial pigmentation.
- Early Kaposi's sarcoma.
- Amalgam tattoo.
- Naevi.
- Melanotic macule.
- Pigmentary incontinence.
- Drug induced pigmentation.

Clinical investigation
- Provided that the diagnosis is clear, investigations are not usually required. There may be a history of trauma during restorative dental procedures, or extraction of a heavily restored tooth.
- Where there is doubt as to the diagnosis, biopsy should be undertaken.
- Radiographs may reveal sizeable particles of amalgam or other radiopaque material, but small particulate matter will not be shown radiologically.

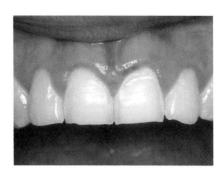

Fig 3-22 A gingival ephelis.

Management options
- Dental amalgam is usually well-tolerated and no active intervention is required.
- The patient should be reassured as to the nature of the condition.

In addition to amalgam tattoos, blue/black pigmentation of the marginal gingivae may occur as a result of adjacent ceramo-metallic crowns. This is again due to metal salts leaching out of the metallic superstructure of the restoration.

Melanotic Macule (Ephelis)
Clinical features
- Small, pale brown, flat areas of pigmentation that are uncommonly seen on the gingivae (Fig 3-22).
- Asymptomatic.
- They do not usually enlarge nor darken with time.
- Present in one per 1000 of the population (all intra-oral sites).
- More common in females (female:male ratio – 2:1).

Aetiology
- Obscure.

Involvement of non-gingival sites
- Melanotic macules are more frequently seen at other sites such as the lips, palate or the skin, where they may accompany the ageing process.

Differential diagnosis
- Racial pigmentation.
- Early Kaposi's sarcoma.

- Naevi.
- Pigmentary incontinence.
- Smoker's melanosis.
- Drug induced pigmentation.

Clinical investigation
- Biopsy if there is doubt as to the nature of the lesion.

Management options
- No active intervention is required.
- Patient reassurance.

Naevi
Intra oral naevi are uncommon and particularly so on the gingivae.

Clinical features
- Range in colour from blue/brown to dark brown.
- They may be flat or papular.
- Their size and colour do not usually change with time.
- Any sudden changes in the clinical appearance should raise suspicion. However the large majority of naevi do not transform to melanoma.
- Naevi are asymptomatic.

Aetiology
- Developmental localised increase in the number of melanocytes.

Involvement of non-gingival sites
- More usually found in the palate and skin.

Differential diagnosis
- Racial pigmentation.
- Early Kaposi's sarcoma.
- Amalgam tattoo.
- Melanotic macule.
- Pigmentary incontinence.
- Drug induced pigmentation.

Clinical investigation
- Excisional biopsy will confirm the diagnosis.

Management options
- Excision biopsy is prudent to exclude sinister pathology.

Malignant Melanoma
Intra-oral malignant melanoma is a rare tumour with a poor prognosis. Median survival is less than two years following diagnosis. The tumour may arise de novo or in approximately 30% cases it will occur within areas of hyperpigmentation. Oral malignant melanomas account for only 1% of total cases of the condition, although in Japanese patients oral involvement accounts for 11% of all melanomas.

Clinical features
- A pigmented lesion demonstrating the following features should arouse suspicion:
  - Dark pigmentation, often varying in intensity over the lesion.
  - Haemorrhage.
  - Crusting.
  - Ulceration.
  - Nodularity.
  - Inflammation.
  - Rapid growth.
  - Satellite areas of pigmentation.
  - Sudden change in the clinical features of a pre-existing pigmented lesion.
- Gingival lesions most frequently involve the maxilla.
- A minority of lesions may initially appear benign. Thus pigmented lesions should always be viewed with an index of suspicion.

Aetiology
- Malignant tumour of melanocytes.
- Exposure to ultraviolet radiation cannot be a significant factor in the development of intra-oral melanoma as it is for cutaneous disease.

Involvement of non-gingival sites
- The palatal mucosa is the most frequently involved intra-oral site. 80% of oral melanomas occur here or on the palatal gingivae (Fig 3-23).
- Sun-exposed skin.
- The tongue and buccal mucosa may be sites of metastatic melanoma deposits.

Differential diagnosis
- Naevus.

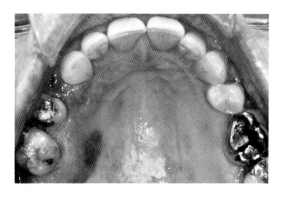

Fig 3-23 Malignant melanoma involving the palatal mucosa.

- Racial pigmentation.
- Kaposi's sarcoma.
- Amalgam tattoo.
- Melanotic macule.
- Addison's disease.
- Pigmentary incontinence.
- Drug induced pigmentation.

Clinical investigation
- Histological confirmation of the diagnosis is mandatory.

Management options
- Wide excision.
- Superficial lesions have a more favourable prognosis.

Further Reading

Reichart PA, Philipsen HP. Oral erythroplakia – a review. Oral Oncology 2005; 41:6,551-561.

Sciubba J. Oral leukoplakia. Critical Reviews in Oral Biology and Medicine 1995; 6:2,147-160.

Rhodus NL. Oral Cancer: leukoplakia and squamous cell carcinoma. Dental Clinics of North America. 2005; 49:1,143-165.

Rugg E, Magee G, Wilson N, Brandrup F, Hamburger J, Lane E. Identification of two novel mutations in keratin 13 as the cause of white sponge naevus. Oral Diseases 1999; 5:4,321-324.

Chapter 4
Gingival Colour Changes – Generalised

Aim

This chapter aims to identify those conditions that may produce widespread colour changes of the gingivae.

Outcome

Having read this chapter, the reader should have a working knowledge of the various conditions that can cause generalised red, white and pigmented areas on the gingivae. Additionally there should be an understanding of the differential diagnoses for these respective conditions, together with an appreciation of the nature of the salient clinical investigations required for a definitive diagnosis and subsequent treatment. Table 4-1 summarises the conditions discussed in the text.

Red Lesions

The most frequent cause of generalised reddening of the gingivae is that of plaque-associated gingivitis. This topic is extensively covered in various other books in this series and therefore will not be addressed in this chapter.

Desquamative Gingivitis

Desquamative gingivitis is a relatively common clinical presentation, particularly in middle aged to elderly female patients. It is a descriptive term and not a diagnosis in itself. It is therefore important to identify the underlying cause of the condition to ensure appropriate patient management.

Clinical appearance
- Desquamative gingivitis may range in severity from a mild generalised redness to a florid, fiery red appearance. The gingivae are shiny, smooth and thinned (atrophic), as a consequence of epithelial desquamation (Fig 4-1).
- In some patients the changes are sporadic rather than confluent affecting only certain gingival sites. It is unclear as to why such localisation occurs.
- Desquamative gingivitis may involve both the free and attached gingivae.

Table 4-1 **Summary table – Generalised gingival colour changes**

Major Categories	Sub Categories	Frequency of Condition	Management Setting
Red lesions	Plaque-associated gingivitis	Very common	Primary care with referral to specialist units if refractory to conventional treatment
	Desquamative gingivitis	Common. Most frequently due to lichen planus, but vesiculobullous diseases may also cause this condition.	Initial phase of stringent oral hygiene and topical anti-inflammatories can be undertaken in primary care. Recalcitrant or vesiculobullous disease should be referred to specialist units
	Primary herpetic gingivostomatitis	Uncommon	Supportive measures and antiviral agents such as aciclovir, which are only of real value if therapy instituted at onset or very early in the course of the disease
	Streptococcal gingivostomatitis	Very rare	Difficulty in diagnosis usually means that such cases will be referred for a specialist opinion
	Orofacial granulomatosis	Uncommon	Requires specialist management for diagnosis and treatment

Major Categories	Sub Categories	Frequency of Condition	Management Setting
	Plasma cell gingivitis	Rare	Specialist referral for diagnosis and identification of the allergen (not always possible)
	Other gingival hypersensitivity reactions	Uncommon	If the causative allergen can be readily identified and avoided there is no need for referral
	Sturge–Weber syndrome	Very rare	Specialist referral required
White lesions	Lichen planus	Common	Recalcitrant lichen planus should be referred to specialist units for diagnostic confirmation, treatment and monitoring
	Leukoplakia	Although leukoplakia is not uncommon, it rarely involves large areas of the gingivae	Specialist referral for biopsy (may require multiple samples) and monitoring
	Candidosis	Very rare	Referral to specialist units for further investiagtions

Major Categories	Sub Categories	Frequency of Condition	Management Setting
Pigmented lesions	Extrinsic staining	Very common	Reassurance in primary care with appropriate advice regarding avoidance of such habits as smoking or betel nut usage.
	Racial pigmentation	Very common	Reassurance in primary care
	Drug-induced/heavy metal pigmentation	Uncommon	Primary care or specialist referral if aetiological agent is not obvious
	Addison's disease	Rare	If this condition is suspected, specialist referral is appropriate

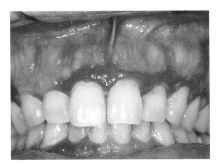
Fig 4-1 Desquamative gingivitis.

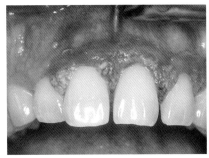
Fig 4-2 Desquamative gingivitis with lichenoid striae.

- Dependent on its aetiology there may be other features, including lichenoid striae, (Fig 4-2) ulceration or rarely vesicle or bulla formation.
- Oral hygiene may be poor in the affected areas, leading to exacerbation of the condition due to superimposed plaque-related gingival inflammation.

Clinical symptoms
- Despite a very florid presentation in some cases, patients can be remarkably free of symptoms.
- It is not uncommon for patients to complain of some degree of soreness, which is heightened by highly flavoured foods and drinks.
- Discomfort may cause difficulties in practising effective oral hygiene measures.

Aetiology
The following conditions may produce a desquamative gingivitis:
- Lichen planus (the most frequent cause – see later).
- Mucous membrane pemphigoid. (See Chapter 8).
- Pemphigus vulgaris. (See Chapter 8).
- Discoid lupus erythematosus.
- Occasionally linear IgA disease.
- Hypersensitivity responses to local allergens including certain components of dentifrices. However, on careful clinical examination, such cases of 'desquamative gingivitis' have a somewhat granular surface appearance rather than the typical smooth appearance described above.
- Historically, the hormonal changes associated with the menopause were considered to be an aetiological factor, in view of the predisposition of menopausal females to present with the condition. There is no substan-

tial evidence for this, the association being more a reflection of the typical age of onset of some of the aetiological factors listed above.

Involvement of non-gingival sites

In many cases there may be no other intra-oral or extra-oral involvement. In other cases examination will reveal lesions consistent with one of the aetiological conditions, such as lichenoid striae on the buccal mucosa.

In mucous membrane pemphigoid and pemphigus, desquamative gingivitis may be the first presenting clinical sign, sometimes predating the occurrence of other features by several years. It is therefore important to ascertain if there is any extra-oral involvement (for example ocular in the case of pemphigoid), so that appropriate therapy can be commenced prior to irreversible tissue damage.

Differential diagnosis

- The aetiological conditions discussed above.
- Orofacial granulomatosis.
- Myeloproliferative disease.
- Linear gingivitis as seen in HIV/AIDS.

Clinical investigation

- Desquamative gingivitis is diagnosed on clinical features.
- Biopsy of gingivae may be diagnostically unhelpful as a result of the non-specific background inflammation masking specific features of the underlying pathology.
- Biopsy of involved oral mucosa (if present) is often more valuable diagnostically.
- Indirect and direct immunofluorescence are indicated if there is a suspicion of an autoimmune vesiculobullous disease. Specimens for direct immunofluorescence studies must be unfixed and transferred to the laboratory as soon as possible for appropriate processing. The specimen should be transported in 'Michel's medium' or wrapped carefully in saline-soaked gauze.

Management options

Desquamative gingivitis is often resistant to effective treatment. A high standard of oral hygiene is an essential prerequisite to improving the condition. Appropriate therapy for the aetiological condition should be implemented and topical corticosteroid therapy may be helpful, particularly if administered under occlusion, e.g. fluocinolone acetonide cream

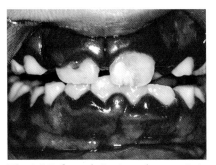 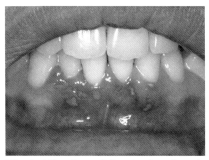

Fig 4-3 Inflamed gingivae characteristic of primary herpetic gingivostomatitis.

Fig 4-4 Erosion of the gingivae in primary herpetic gingivostomatitis.

delivered via a mouthguard to ensure adequate contact with the affected areas.

Primary Herpetic Gingivostomatitis

Most cases of primary herpes simplex infection are subclinical and essentially asymptomatic, the patient sometimes having mild non-specific symptoms of malaise and lymphadenopathy. Approximately 10% of cases will manifest as an acute gingivostomatitis with marked systemic malaise.

Clinical appearance
- Florid, red oedematous gingivae (Fig 4-3).
- Distribution is not plaque related.
- Hypersalivation.
- Vesicles and ulceration of the gingivae, although these are usually present at other oral mucosal sites (Fig 4-4).

Clinical symptoms
- Usually occurs in children although young adults are increasingly affected.
- Acute onset with fever, malaise, sore throat and lymphadenopathy.
  - In young adults the infection can, on occasions, be severe enough to warrant hospital admission and may be confused with Stevens Johnson syndrome.
- Pain from the involved tissues.

Aetiology
- Primary infection is usually due to herpes simplex type 1 virus but HSV type 2 infection may also be involved.

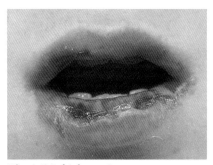

Fig 4-5 Labial crusting.

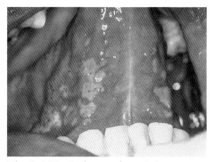

Fig 4-6 Typical ragged serpiginous erosions of Herpes simplex infection.

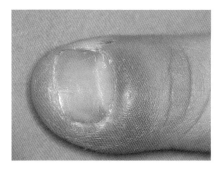

Fig 4-7 Herpetic whitlow.

- Recurrent or secondary infection produces a herpetic cold sore, although in the immunocompromised, it may manifest in a similar fashion to the primary infection.

Involvement of non-gingival sites
- Vesicles that rapidly ulcerate appear on the palate, tongue, buccal mucosa, labial mucosa and vermilion border producing characteristic haemorrhagic crusting of the lips (Fig 4-5).
- The individual ulcers coalesce together forming large serpiginous areas of ulceration covered with a grey/white slough (Fig 4-6).
- Transmission of the virus to other sites such as the nail beds (herpetic whitlow) (Fig 4-7) and the eye (conjunctivitis; keratitis).
- Very rarely encephalitis.

Differential diagnosis
- Erythema multiforme.
- Myeloproliferative disease.
- Myelosuppressive disease.

Clinical investigation
- The diagnosis is usually made on clinical grounds.
- Viral identification in vesicle fluid.
- Demonstration of a rising serum antibody titre in sequential paired blood samples (i.e. acute and convalescent antibody titres).
- Immunofluorescence to identify specific serum IgM antibodies in a single blood sample (i.e. evidence of a primary immune response).

Management options
- Supportive measures (fluids, anti-inflammatories, rest).
- Aciclovir administered early in the course of the disease (ideally before vesiculation).
- Avoid disseminating the infection to other sites (i.e. by avoiding scratching or picking the oral lesions).

Streptococcal Gingivostomatitis
This is a very rare condition and may cause diagnostic confusion with viral infections, particularly primary herpetic gingivostomatitis. It may manifest in children or young adults, producing widespread inflammation and soreness of the gingivae and oral mucosa. Ulceration may also occur, but there is no vesiculation, an important diagnostic feature that helps differentiate this infection from those with a viral aetiology. The diagnosis can be confirmed by identifying Group A beta-haemolytic streptococci in culture. The infection is usually susceptible to treatment with penicillin (Katz, 2002).

Orofacial Granulomatosis
Orofacial granulomatosis may involve the gingivae by producing generalised band like inflammatory change that is not plaque-related and extends across the width of the attached gingivae and on to the alveolar mucosa (Fig 4-8). Additionally the condition may also produce a generalised gingival overgrowth. A full account of orofacial granulomatosis can be found in Chapter 6.

Plasma Cell Gingivitis
Clinical appearance
- Plasma cell gingivitis is an unusual condition that produces a diffuse, reddened somewhat granular appearance to the affected gingivae (Fig 4-9).

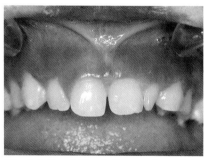

Fig 4-8 Band-like inflammation of the attached gingivae and alveolar mucosa in orofacial granulomatosis.

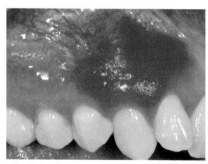

Fig 4-9 Plasma cell gingivitis.

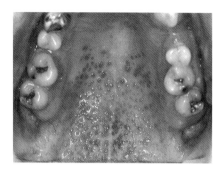

Fig 4-10 Plasma cell stomatitis involving the palate and oropharynx.

- It may be confused with desquamative gingivitis.

Clinical symptoms
- Patients may complain of soreness but often the condition is asymptomatic.

Aetiology
- The condition appears to be related to hypersensitivity responses to a variety of potential allergens including:
  - Additives to dentifrices e.g. cinnamonaldehyde or sodium lauryl sulphate.
  - Food additives and flavouring agents.
  - Dental materials.
  - Essential oils including eugenol.
  - Drugs.
  - Mouthwashes.

Involvement of non-gingival sites
• Plasma cell stomatitis is a very rare condition but may involve any part of the oral mucosa including the palate and oropharynx (Fig 4-10).

Differential diagnosis
• Plaque associated gingivitis/periodontitis.
• Desquamative gingivitis.
• Orofacial granulomatosis.
• Kaposi's sarcoma.
• Primary herpetic gingivistomatitis.

Clinical investigation
• Diagnosis is usually made on clinical grounds.
• Skin testing for potential allergens may sometimes be helpful but often this is not the case.
• Biopsy.

Management options
• Identification and avoidance of the causative allergen.
• Corticosteroids may also be helpful in suppressing the inflammatory response.

Other hypersensitivity reactions of the gingivae
Not all hypersensitivity reactions that occur within the gingivae manifest as a plasma cell gingivitis. There may be a non-specific reddening of the gingivae, which may be swollen and slightly granular in appearance. This may mimic plaque-associated gingivitis, desquamative gingivitis, or the gingival changes seen in some patients with orofacial granulomatosis or HIV disease.

Allergens that may provoke such reactions are diverse and may include some of the components of dentifrices, mouthwashes, dietary allergens such as food additives and dental materials. The mechanism may be that of a contact sensitivity or less frequently an immediate-type hypersensitivity. Management involves identification of the allergen (not always easy to achieve) and its avoidance in the future.

Occasionally direct chemical toxicity rather than an immunologically mediated reaction may produce a similar clinical presentation (Fig 4-11).

Sturge Weber Syndrome
Sturge Weber syndrome is a rare, congenital, hamartomatous condition

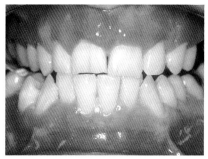

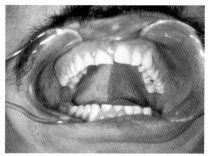

Fig 4-11 Local toxicity due to formaldehyde-containing desensitising dentifrice.

Fig 4-12 Sturge Weber syndrome – intra-oral involvement.

manifesting as angiomas that typically involve those tissues innervated by the trigeminal nerve. Intracranial involvement also occurs, including haemangiomata and calcification of the leptomeninges potentially resulting in learning difficulties and epilepsy.

Clinical features
- The haemangiomata are usually unilateral involving the facial skin, gingivae and oral mucosa (Fig 4-12).
- The lesions are usually flat and red/purple in colour, typical of vascular lesions.
- Occasionally the involved gingivae may appear hyperplastic.

Differential diagnosis
- Other causes of vascular anomalies.

Clinical investigation
- Imaging techniques including Doppler ultrasound and Magnetic Resonance Imaging are of value in defining the location and extent of the lesions.

Management options
- The haemangiomata may pose a potential problem in patients undergoing oral surgical procedures.
- The hemangiomata are only treated if they are causing specific clinical problems.

White Lesions

Lichen Planus (see also Chapter 8)

Lichen planus is a relatively common mucocutaneous inflammatory condition, affecting approximately 2% of the population. It has a female predilection and its onset is typically in middle age and later life. The condition is particularly persistent in the mouth, lasting for many years (10-20 years), and this contrasts with the cutaneous lesions, which often, but not always, resolve after two to three years. The clinical course of lichen planus is generally benign, but a small number of cases may undergo malignant transformation (0.1-1%). This is considered to be more likely in the erosive or atrophic variants.

Clinical appearance
- Lichen planus affecting the gingivae may present as a desquamative gingivitis or with the typical lacy network of non-ulcerating white lichenoid striae, often set on an erythematous base. (Fig 4-13).
- Lichen planus may manifest in other clinical variants including erosive, atrophic, plaque-like and rarely bullous forms.
- Lichen planus is the most frequent cause of desquamative gingivitis.
- Erosive lesions on the gingivae, for example when associated with a desquamative gingivitis should raise suspicion of a vesiculobullous disorder rather than lichen planus itself.
- Desquamative gingivitis may appear fiery red. Plaque accumulation further exacerbates this condition.
- Lesions may be widespread and are classically, but not universally, bilateral and often symmetrical.
- Gingival involvement is common, occurring in up to 30%-50% of affected patients and it may be the only site of involvement (Fig 4-14).
- Pigmentary incontinence may be seen in some cases, particularly in dark-skinned races (Fig 4-15).

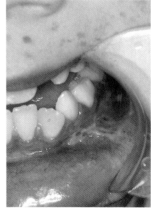

Clinical symptoms
- Patients with reticular lichen planus are asymptomatic or may complain of roughness of the gums.

Fig 4-13 Lichen planus manifesting as desquamative gingivitis with lichenoid striae.

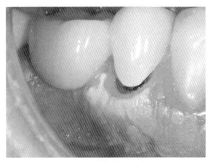

Fig 4-14 Gingival lichen planus.

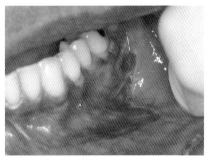

Fig 4-15 Pigmentary incontinence in long standing oral lichen planus.

- Patients with atrophic or desquamative gingivitis experience varying levels of discomfort, which can be severe. This may cause difficulty with effective oral hygiene measures.

Aetiology
- The aetiology of lichen planus is poorly understood.
- Its pathogenesis appears to be T-cell dependent (Sugarman, 2002).
- It is weakly associated with autoimmune liver disease such as Primary Biliary Cirrhosis and Chronic Active Hepatitis.
- Lesions resembling those of lichen planus (lichenoid lesions) are seen in:
  - Chronic Graft Versus Host Disease following bone marrow transplantation (Figs 4-16 and 4-17).
  - As a consequence of a large number of medications (e.g. non-steroidal anti-inflammatory drugs, β-blockers, gold.)
  - Occupational exposure to phenolphthalein dyes in the photographic industry.
  - Mercury amalgam sensitivity (and possibly some composite resin restorative materials).
  - Hepatitis C in certain populations, e.g. Japanese, Italians. However, this may reflect background carriage rate rather than being of aetiological significance.

Involvement of non-gingival sites
- Classically oral lichen planus is a bilaterally symmetrical eruption affecting the buccal mucosae, distally and rarely extends as far as the anterior commissures. (Figs 4-18 and 4-19).

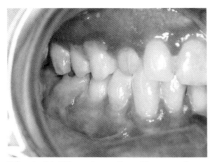

Fig 4-16 Chronic oral graft versus host disease (GvHD) following stem cell transplant for aplastic anaemia, showing a desquamative gingivitis.

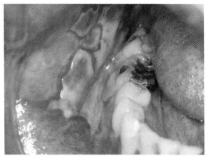

Fig 4-17 GvHD in the same patient as Fig 4-16 showing extensive oral ulceration.

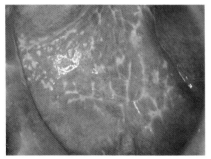

Fig 4-18 Reticular lichen planus of the buccal mucosa.

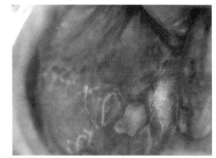

Fig 4-19 Erosive lichen planus of the buccal mucosa.

- The lateral and ventral surfaces of the tongue are also frequently involved (Fig 4-20).
- Any other intra-oral site may also be involved, although the palate and lips are usually spared.
- Cutaneous involvement may occur in 10-30% of patients with oral lesions. This typically affects the flexor surfaces of the limbs and wrists, presenting as 'purple polygonal pruritic papules' with the classical white Wickham's striae running through them (Fig 4-21). As in the mouth, lesions are often bilaterally symmetrical.
- Other mucosal surfaces may also be involved such as the genitalia. In females, involvement of the vulva and vagina together with a desquamative gingivitis is known as the 'vulvo-vaginal gingival syndrome'.
- The scalp may also be affected.

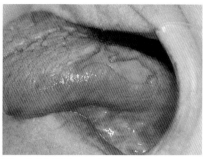 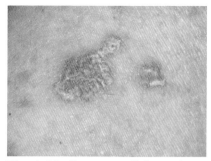

Fig 4-20 Lichen planus of the tongue, showing a typical atrophic appearance.

Fig 4-21 Cutaneous lichen planus showing the classical papular eruption

Differential diagnosis
- Drug-induced lichenoid eruptions.
- Lichenoid eruptions secondary to dental restorations.
- Discoid/systemic lupus erythematosus.
- Mucous membrane pemphigoid.
- Pemphigus.
- Graft versus host disease.
- Leukoplakia.
- Plasma cell gingivitis.
- Chronic hyperplastic candidosis.
- Squamous cell carcinoma.
- Non-specific ulceration.
- Hairy leukoplakia.

Clinical investigation
- Biopsy if there is doubt clinically as to the diagnosis of non-erosive lesions.
- Biopsy erosive/atrophic lesions to confirm the diagnosis and identify possible dysplasia.
- Smear for candidal organisms.
- Investigate for underlying disease if suspected clinically.

Management options
In asymptomatic cases there is no need for active treatment. In symptomatic cases, the aim is to reduce inflammation and heal erosions. Oral lichen planus is very persistent and curative treatment is as yet unavailable. Treatment should be via a stepped approach, using topical therapy whenever possible.

- Ensure excellent oral hygiene.
- Identification and substitution of associated drug if appropriate.
- Consider removal of amalgam restorations if there is a suspicion that they may be contributory.
- Treatment of an identifiable underlying disease.
- Topical agents:
  - Chlorhexidine as an adjunct to oral hygiene measures
  - Corticosteroids – e.g. soluble prednisolone, soluble betamethasone, beclometasone, fluticasone propionate.
  - Fluocinolone may be particularly helpful in desquamative gingivitis when administered under occlusion via a mouthguard.
- Intralesional corticosteroids – triamcinolone acetonide
- Systemic corticosteroids – prednisolone, deflazacort. Steroid sparing agents such as azathioprine may also be considered.
- In particularly recalcitrant cases, topical ciclosporin or tacrolimus may be used. However caution is needed with the prescription of these drugs, which are best used in specialist units to ensure appropriate monitoring. There are currently concerns regarding possible carcinogenicity associated with the use of topical tacrolimus. Its usage must therefore be restricted to very severe cases, when it should only be used for a limited duration.
- Long-term follow up is mandatory for atrophic and erosive variants due to the possibility (albeit small) of malignant transformation.

Other Generalised White Lesions
Gingival candidosis and leukoplakia may be widespread in their distribution on occasions, although more usually present as discrete areas of colour change.

Pigmented Lesions

Extrinsic Staining
Staining of the gingivae may also occur as a consequence of various local agents, including the consumption of highly coloured foods and drink and the use of betel nut.

Betel nut is used by a variety of Asian communities and produces a characteristic brown/orange staining of the oral mucosa, gingivae and teeth (Fig 4-22).

Heavy tobacco consumption may also produce extrinsic staining of the tissues but additionally it also causes intrinsic melanosis.

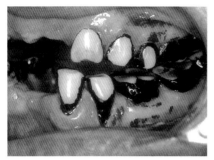 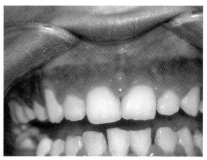

Fig 4-22 Extrinsic staining due to chewing betel nut.

Fig 4-23 Racial pigmentation of the gingivae.

Racial Pigmentation
Clinical Features
- Diffuse macular brown areas, often widespread (Fig 4-23).
- Frequently associated with the anterior labial gingivae.
- Common in dark-skinned populations – Asian and Afro-Caribbean individuals.

Involvement of non-gingival sites
- Pigmentation may occur at any intra-oral site.
- The dorsum of tongue and buccal mucosa are frequently involved.

Differential diagnosis
- Pigmentary incontinence secondary to chronic inflammatory disease of the oral mucosa.
- Smoker's melanosis.
- Addison's disease.
- Pregnancy.
- Melanotic macules.
- Drug-induced pigmentation.
- HIV/AIDS.
- Peutz–Jegher syndrome.
- Laugier-Hunziker syndrome.

Clinical investigation
- Exclusion of other causes of generalised gingival pigmentation (consider investigations for Addison's disease – see below)

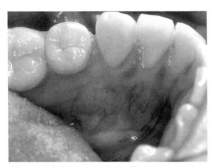 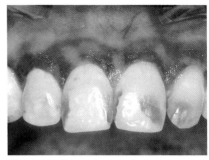

Fig 4-24 Drug-induced pigmentation due to minocycline.

Fig 4-25 Drug-induced pigmentation due to AZT.

Management options
• No active intervention is required other than reassurance.

Drug-Induced and Heavy Metal Pigmentation
A variety of drugs and also heavy metals can produce diffuse gingival discolouration.

It is therefore important to take a detailed medical history for patients, noting the patient's systemic medication.

Additionally it is important to consider possible occupational exposure to heavy metals, although this is now uncommon due to improved health and safety regulations that are intended to limit such exposure.

The discolouration will vary according to the causative agent:
• For example, minocycline can cause a purple/grey discoloration (Fig 4-24), whilst other drugs such as cytotoxics and AZT (Fig 4-25), may lead to brown pigmentation.

Some of the more commonly used drugs associated with mucosal discolouration are listed below:
• Anticonvulsants. e.g. phenytoin.
• Antimalarials.
• ACTH.
• The oral contraceptive pill.
• Antimicrobials including minocycline, ketoconazole, zidovudine and clofazimine.

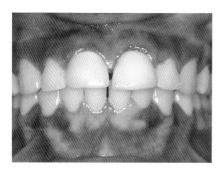

Fig 4-26 Diffuse gingival pigmentation as a result of Addison's disease.

- Cytotoxic drugs including busulphan and cyclophosphamide.
- Amiodarone.
- Chlorpromazine.

Heavy metals associated with mucosal discolouration include:
- Arsenic.
- Bismuth.
- Copper.
- Gold.
- Lead.
- Mercury.
- Platinum.
- Silver.
- Zinc.

Addison's Disease
Addison's disease is a rare condition occurring more frequently in females. It results from the destruction (usually autoimmune) of the adrenal cortex.

Clinical appearance
- Diffuse brown pigmentation of the gingivae (Fig 4-26).

Clinical symptoms
- Oral manifestations are asymptomatic.
- Systemically there is often vague symptomatology of lethargy, malaise, weakness, anorexia or vomiting.
- Fainting as a result of postural hypotension.

Aetiology
- 90% of cases are autoimmune (21-hydroxylase being the usual antigen).
- Excessive production of adrenocortictrophic hormone (ACTH) in response to low serum cortisol levels produces hyperpigmentation as a consequence of certain of its properties being similar to those of melanocyte stimulating hormone.

Involvement of non-gingival sites
- There may be increased pigmentation at cutaneous and other mucosal sites such as the genitalia.
- Cutaneous hyperpigmentation is seen especially within skin creases.

Differential diagnosis
- Racial pigmentation.
- Drug-induced pigmentation.
- Smoker's melanosis.
- Pregnancy.
- Malignant melanoma.
- Melanotic macules.

Clinical investigation
- Isolated plasma cortisol levels are of little value.
- In suspected Addison's disease, preliminary investigations that may be undertaken include the following:
  - Blood pressure recording, which may be hypotensive.
  - Plasma electrolytes may demonstrate hyponatraemia and hyperkalaemia.
  - Serum urea may be elevated.
  - Blood glucose level may be depressed.
- Definitive investigation is afforded by an ACTH stimulation test.

Management options
- The hyperpigmented lesions do not require treatment.
- Recognition of the possible underlying diagnosis is important with referral to the appropriate specialty for diagnostic confirmation.
- Glucocorticoid and mineralocorticoid replacement by the appropriate physician.

Further Reading

Katz J, Guelmann M, Rudolph M, Ruskin J. Acute streptococcal infection of the gingiva, lower lip and pharynx – a case report. Journal of Periodontology 2002; 73:11,1392-1395.

Sugarman PB, Savage NW, Walsh LJ et al. The pathogenesis of oral lichen planus. Critical Reviews in Oral Biology and Medicine 2002; 13:4,350-365.

Chapter 5
Gingival Enlargements – Localised

Aim

This chapter aims to provide the practitioner with a visual guide to swellings that arise locally within the gingiva, including the free and/or attached gingiva.

Outcome

At the end of this chapter the reader should have knowledge of which types of localised gingival swellings are common or uncommon, be able to identify the key clinical features of localised gingival enlargements and formulate a differential diagnosis for a localised gingival swelling. The reader will also be able to decide which lesions can be managed within their practice and which need to be referred for specialist advice.

Table 5-1 lists the gingival enlargements discussed in this chapter and highlights which are common or uncommon and when the condition may be managed in general practice or should be referred.

The Epulides

Gingival epulides are benign localised enlargements of the gingival tissues. They are predominantly hyperplastic lesions of the gingival connective tissues, which develop following chronic irritation. The source of irritation may vary and examples include:
• Ledged or prominent subgingival restorations.
• Subgingival calculus.
• Clasp arms from removable appliances.
• Impaction of a foreign body subgingivally.

Many lesions may present as epulides, but only three true forms are described:
• Fibrous epulis.
• Vascular epulis (pyogenic granuloma or pregnancy epulis).
• Giant cell epulides (peripheral or centrally arising).

Table 5-1 **Localised gingival swellings**

Lesions	Category	Sub-Category	Incidence	Manage/Refer
True epulides	Fibrous epulis		common (60% of epulides)	manage
	Vascular epulis	Pyogenic granuloma Pregnancy epulis	common (30% of epulides)	manage
		Multiple/disseminated pyogenic granuloma	uncommon	refer
	Giant cell epulis/ granuloma	Peripheral	uncommon (10%)	refer
		Central	uncommon	refer
Lesions presenting as epulides	Congenital epulis		uncommon	refer
	Viral warts	Condyloma acuminatum	uncommon	refer
		Verruca vulgaris	uncommon	refer
	Neurofibroma		uncommon	refer
	Appliance-induced hyperplasia		common	manage

Lesions	Category	Sub-Category	Incidence	Manage/Refer
Other gingival swellings	Abscess	Periodontal	common	manage
		Gingival	uncommon	manage
		Stitch	uncommon	manage
	Localised trauma		uncommon	manage/refer
	Histiocytosis-X	Unifocal (solitary eosinophilic granuloma)	uncommon	refer
		Multifocal (Hand–Schuller–Christian syndrome)		
		Progressive/disseminated (Letterer–Siwe disease)		
	Haemangioma		uncommon	refer
Tumours	Malignant lesions	Kaposi's sarcoma	uncommon	refer
		Squamous cell carcinoma	uncommon	refer
		Metastatic tumours	uncommon	refer
		Non-Hodgkin's lymphoma	uncommon	refer
	Benign lesions	Reactive osteoma	uncommon	manage
	Lesions associated with PTEN mutations	Cowden's syndrome	uncommon	refer
		Bannayan–Riley–Ruvalcaba syndrome		
		Proteus syndrome		

The term epulis means 'on the gum', and all true epulides have a common pathogenesis, which involves the body attempting to heal an area of inflammation through the formation of granulation and fibrous tissue, whilst the inflammatory stimulus remains. Therefore, true epulides are histologically similar and show variable features of chronic inflammation, immature vascular tissue (granulation tissue) and collagen deposition. The only exception is the congenital epulis.

The Fibrous Epulis
Clinical appearance
Fibrous epulides present as pink, firm enlargements of the interdental gingivae (Fig 5-1). They may be sessile or pedunculated and similar in colour to the surrounding tissues unless they become inflamed. Ulceration can arise, leading to a yellow, fibrinous surface exudate. They are normally firm in consistency, do not blanch, and pitting of the surface may be seen due to the insertion of collagen bundles beneath. Calcification or ossification may arise within some lesions, when the term 'calcifying or cementifying fibrous epulis' is used. The behaviour and treatment of the latter is the same, but recurrence is reported to be more common.

Clinical symptoms
Often symptom-free and predominantly cause aesthetic concerns. Rarely they can lead to tooth migration and irritation to the overlying soft tissues (e.g. lip).

Aetiology
As for all epulides (see previous text).

Involvement of non-gingival sites
None.

Differential diagnosis
- Vascular epulis.
- Giant cell granuloma.
- Benign osteoma of underlying alveolar bone.
- Denture induced hyperplasia.
- Gingival cyst.
- Neurofibroma.
- Connective tissue tumour (see chapter 11).
- Metastatic tumour.

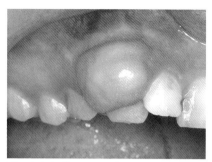 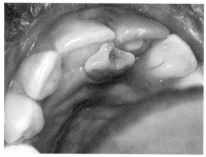

Fig 5-1 A fibrous epulis UR 3 related to chronic irritation from subgingival calculus acting as a plaque retention factor.

Fig 5-2 A pregnancy epulis affecting UR1 and UL1 teeth and demonstrating a classical dumb-bell or hourglass shape between the incisors.

Clinical investigation

Excisional biopsy for histopathology with careful gingival recontouring. Lesions consists of a core of highly cellular fibroblastic and granulation tissue covered by stratified squamous epithelium, which may or may not be ulcerated. There are varying degrees of inflammatory cell infiltration, mainly with plasma cells.

Management options

If large, referral is advisable. Surgical excision followed by recontouring of the gingivae to form a marginal complex that lends itself to easy cleansing. Thorough subgingival debridement is performed to remove potential aetiological agents, e.g. calculus, foreign body, plaque. Apply a pressure pack, to maintain the interproximal zone patent during the healing phase. Chlorhexidine mouthwash is advisable during this period, and the patient should be reviewed after seven days for dressing removal and prophylaxis. At this stage the patient should resume careful interproximal plaque control. Lesions may recur if the cause of the irritation persists.

The Vascular Epulis
Clinical appearance

Vascular epulides mainly arise in the anterior part of the mouth and usually, the labial aspect. They are soft, normally pedunculated lesions with a narrow base which, when associated with pregnancy (Fig 5-2), can progress throughout the gestation period. Commonly they occur in the second or third trimester and may have a very red/granular surface that is prone to haemorrhage (spontaneous or as a result of trauma). The surface may ulcerate, leaving a yellow, fibrinous coating (Fig 5-3).

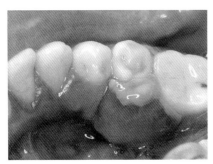 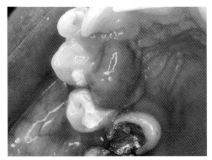

Fig 5-3 A vascular epulis affecting LR5. The surface has ulcerated due to trauma from the opposing teeth.

Fig 5-4 A pyogenic granuloma (vascular epulis) arising UR45 area due to poorly contoured subgingival temporary dressings.

Clinical symptoms
Bleeding to touch or when brushing, poor aesthetics and discomfort on pressure.

Aetiology
The pregnancy epulis and pyogenic granuloma (Fig 5-4) are histologically identical. The term 'pyogenic granuloma' is a historical one, since it was thought (incorrectly) that the lesion was an inflammatory response to infection with pyogenic bacteria. Lesions develop for the same reasons as other epulides, but vascular changes characterise the inflammatory response rather than fibrosis. Pregnancy-associated lesions are generally associated with subgingival plaque or calculus.

Involvement of non-gingival sites
None.

Differential diagnosis
• Giant cell granuloma.
• Denture induced hyperplasia.
• Fibrous epulis.
• Kaposi's sarcoma.
• Gingival cyst.

Clinical investigation
Presumptive diagnosis can be made on appearance, but definitive diagnosis requires an excision biopsy. Lesions comprise a mass of vascular spaces within

a fine, connective tissue stroma. There may be solid layers of uncanalised endothelium or many thin-walled immature vessels and the surface is often ulcerated, with an inflammatory infiltrate beneath the ulceration. Histologically, the pregnancy epulis is regarded as a pyogenic granuloma arising during pregnancy.

Management options
Intensive oral hygiene instruction and scaling under local anaesthesia reduces the vascular of the lesion and may lead to its resolution. However, excision is often necessary and recurrence rates are high. Good vasoconstriction is essential from a local anaesthetic and an electrosurgery or bi-polar diathermy should be on hand. The area should be thoroughly scaled and a pressure dressing applied. It is common for the lesion to return, therefore excision is preferable post-parturition. Many resolve spontaneously postpartum. The non-pregnancy associated pyogenic granuloma is excised in a similar manner. However, the cause, such as defective restorations, should be identified and removed.

Multiple/Disseminated Pyogenic Granulomata
Clinical appearance
This is an extremely rare condition. The case shown in Figs 5-5 and 5-6 presented in a seven-year-old boy. Appearance is of multiple vascular exophytic lesions, which present as disseminated vascular tumours with a relatively short natural history. Lesions have a fibrinous exudate at their surface, similar to solitary pyogenic granulomas. Satellite and intravenous pyogenic gran-

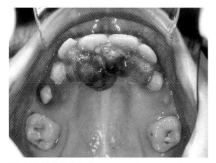

Fig 5-5 Multiple pyogenic granulomas in a seven-year-old boy affecting the palatal aspects of his anterior teeth.

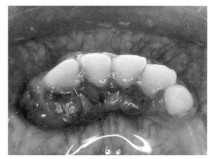

Fig 5-6 The same boy as in Fig 5-5 with multiple lesions affecting the lower incisor teeth.

ulomas may develop at the same time as the primary lesion or may occur after attempted treatment of the primary lesion. Lesions may be grouped or eruptive and disseminated in nature.

Clinical symptoms
There is gingival bleeding when the tissues are subject to light trauma from brushing or eating. Spontaneous bleeding is also reported.

Aetiology
Trauma, hormonal influences, viral oncogenes, underlying microscopic arteriovenous malformations, and production of angiogenic factors have all been implicated. However, in the case illustrated, the likely aetiology was of oral neglect and local irritation or trauma causing a primary lesion, which then spread laterally.

Involvement of non-gingival sites
A space occupying lesion between the fifth and eighth thoracic vertebrae was identified by MRI scan in this case, which led to a spastic diplegic gait and lower limb paralysis. There was also weight loss and chronic diarrhoea. Syringomyelia was diagnosed (a disorder in which a cyst forms within the spinal cord). This cyst, called a syrinx, expands and elongates over time, destroying the centre of the cord. Damage may result in pain, weakness and stiffness in the legs. Other symptoms include headaches and incontinence.

Differential diagnosis
• Bacillary angiomatosis.
• Benign lymphangioendothelioma.
• Kaposi's sarcoma.
• Leukaemia.
• Kaposiform hemangioendothelioma.

Clinical investigation
Excision biopsy. Histology is identical to the solitary pyogenic granuloma. Whether the spinal cord lesion was a satellite granuloma or a co-incidental true syrinx in this case remains uncertain.

Management options
Specialist referral is essential. Intensive oral hygiene and full mouth prophylaxis restored gingival health in the reported case, and intensive physiotherapy restored lower limb function. Excision of the multiple granulomas, scal-

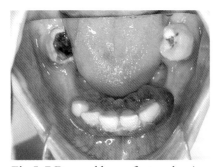

Fig 5-7 Decayed lower first molars in a neglected mouth from the patient illustrated in Figs 5-5 and 5-6, which were extracted to restore oral health.

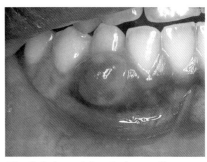

Fig 5-8 A peripheral giant cell granuloma affecting LR 234 teeth.

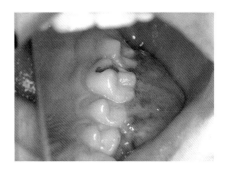

Fig 5-9 A central giant cell lesion that has expanded in the left maxillary premolar and molar region. Note the pigmentation due to haemosiderin deposition.

ing and restoration of high standards of plaque control will help restore oral health (Fig 5-7).

The Giant Cell Epulis

Clinical appearance

This is a pedunculated or sessile lesion, dark red in colour and often with an ulcerated surface (Fig 5-8). Size varies, and lesions may project from palatal through to labial gingivae with a narrow pedicle between the teeth (hourglass appearance). Radiographs are essential, as giant cell epulides may arise centrally within bone as central giant cell granulomas, perforating the outer bone cortex to present peripherally. Lesions may become very large (Fig 5-9) and, unless correctly diagnosed, incomplete excision is likely. Lesions may also arise in association with implants (Fig 5-10).

Clinical symptoms

These usually present between 30-40 years, but also in the very young or

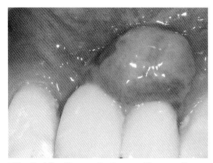

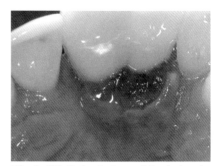

Fig 5-10a Central giant cell granuloma arising around implant fixtures UL1 and 2, which were placed into an autogenous bone graft (from the right chin). The lesion had been excised unsuccessfully three times at presentation.

Fig 5-10b Palatal view of the lesion in 5-10a.

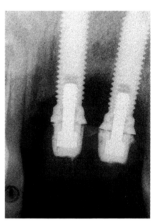

Fig 5-10c Bone loss associated with central giant cell granuloma in Fig 5-10a and b. The implant fixtures had to be removed prior to aggressive curettage of the surrounding bone.

old, whether dentate or edentulous. They are most common in the anterior region of the mouth and twice as common in females as males. They are more prevalent in the mandible than the maxilla, and symptoms include bleeding to touch or when brushing, poor aesthetics and discomfort on pressure.

Aetiology
Aetiology is unknown and, like the other true epulides, is believed to be a reactive hyperplasia due to chronic irritation or trauma. The tissue is thought to be of periosteal origin, but the origin of the giant cells is unknown.

Involvement of non-gingival sites
None, unless arising centrally within bone.

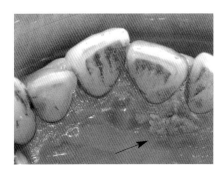

Fig 5-11 A condyloma acuminatum in an HIV patient who had discontinued HAART and was immunosuppressed. Note the adjacent secondary lesion.

Differential diagnosis
• Vascular epulis.
• Denture induced hyperplasia.
• Haemangioma.
• Kaposi's sarcoma.
• Gingival cyst.

Clinical investigation
Periapical radiographs are employed to determine whether there is bony involvement/cortical plate erosion. Histopathology is characterised by focal collections of osteoclast-like giant cells of varying size and number. Giant cells are separated by a fibrous connective tissue stroma within which are vascular channels of varying diameter. Extravasated blood cells and haemosiderin may add a brown/red colour to the lesion (Chapter 4). Bony trabeculae or osteoid (bone matrix) may also be present.

Management options
Excision as for a vascular epulis or if central bone involvement is suspected, a mucoperiosteal flap should be raised and the bone surface curetted. If the gingival margin is involved (e.g. Fig 5-1), care should be taken not to deform the marginal tissues during excision.

Congenital Epulis
This very rarely arises in the anterior maxilla or mandible of newborn children. Its aetiology is unknown, but it is thought to be reactive. It is benign and does not recur following excision.

Viral 'Wart-like' Lesions
Clinical appearance
• Condyloma acuminatum (Ca) (Fig 5-11 and 5-12) is usually present in

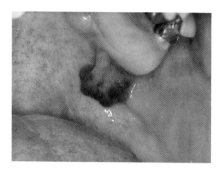

Fig 5-12 A condyloma acuminatum on the right maxillary tuberosity.

immunosuppressed patients and has a 1.2% incidence in HIV disease. There are mushroom-like warts, usually pedunculated. It is contagious and may spread locally.

- Verruca vulgaris (Vv) may be seen on the lips of children with finger warts and appear like small cauliflowers with white-tipped surface papillary projections. It is highly contagious and may spread to other sites of the body.
- Focal epithelial hyperplasia (Heck's disease) is caused by the human papilloma virus (HPV) but does not usually involve the gingivae.
- Molluscum contageosum may present as a localised red lesion, with a granular appearance to its surface.

Clinical symptoms
- Ca – Irritation to the tongue and appearance may cause concern.
- Vv – Roughness to the touch and appearance may be a concern.
- Focal epithelial hyperplasia (FEH) – multiple lumps/roughness.
- Molluscum contageosum produce localised aesthetic problems and may spread from or to the skin.

Aetiology
- Ca – human papilloma virus (HPV) types 6, 11, 16, 18.
- Vv – HPV types 2, 4, 40, 57.
- FEH – over 70 types of HPV have been identified to date.
- Molluscum contageosum is caused by a poxvirus related to smallpox.

Involvement of non-gingival sites
- Ca – Anal or genital involvement.
- Vv – Lesions usually affect the skin of the fingers.
- FEH – Lesions affect oral mucosa generally.
- Molluscum contageosum – commonly affects skin.

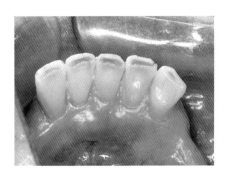

Fig 5-13 A gingival neurofibroma lingual to the lower central incisors.

Differential diagnosis
• Vascular epulis.
• Neurofibromatosis.

Clinical investigation
Presumptive diagnosis is made from clinical findings and following a careful history (including other lesion sites e.g. genitals) and examination of the skin, fingers etc.

Management
Excision or cryosurgery. In HIV disease, lesions may resolve when the patient commences highly active anti-retroviral therapy (HAART).

Neurofibroma
Clinical appearance
Solitary lesions may arise but normally form part of the condition Neurofibromatosis, which may be of type 1 (NF1 or von Recklinghausen's disease - 90% of cases) or type 2 (NF2 – or bilateral acoustic neuromas/schwannomas i.e. higher incidence of central nervous system tumours than NF1). They form well-circumscribed firm focal swellings (Fig 5-13).

Clinical symptoms
These involve largely aesthetic concerns, particularly when multiple skin lesions are present. Neurofibromas present in young adults and increase in number with advancing age.

Aetiology
This is a genetic disorder with no race/sex predilection and an incidence of

one new case in every 3000 live births. The lesions are benign and complex and arise from peripheral nerve sheaths.

Involvement of non-gingival sites
Multiple skin lesions are common and pale brown pigmented patches on the skin, known as café–au–lait spots, may be evident. Multi-organ involvement may arise, including bladder, heart, intestines, kidney and larynx.

Differential diagnosis
If solitary it may appear like:
• fibrous epulis.
• lipoma.
• fibroma.
• reactive osteoma.

Clinical investigation
Biopsy.

Management
Excision if the condition is causing symptoms (aesthetics or functional problems). If multiple, medical management is essential. There is rarely malignant transformation to malignant peripheral nerve sheath tumours or sarcomas.

Dental Appliance-Induced Hyperplasia
Clinical appearance
There is localised gingival enlargement related to chronic irritation from a clasp arm or prosthetic/orthodontic appliance component (Fig 5-14). Ulceration may precede fibrosis (Fig 5-15).

Clinical symptoms
Often there are none, except aesthetic concerns or bleeding when traumatised.

Aetiology
Lesions directly related to irritation by appliance components are caused by a chronic inflammatory reaction, which leads to fibrovascular hyperplasia.

Involvement of non-gingival sites
Lesions arising elsewhere on the oral mucosa are termed fibro-epithelial polyps (Fig 5-16) and are also caused by chronic irritation/trauma.

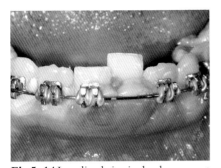

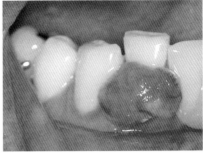

Fig 5-14 Localised gingival enlargement caused by plaque accumulation around a fixed orthodontic appliance LL12. Plaque control was inhibited and the marginal gingivae irritated due to encroachment of the brackets on the gingival margin.

Fig 5-15 Fibrous epulis LR23 with surface ulceration, associated with a poorly fitting lower acrylic partial denture, which has replaced LR1 and LL1.

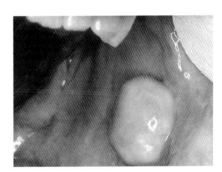

Fig 5-16 A fibroepithelial polyp of the left buccal mucosa caused by chronic trauma from an upper complete denture.

Differential diagnosis
• Fibrous epulis.
• Vascular epulis.

Clinical investigation
Excisional biopsy shows fibro-epithelial hyperplasia with chronic inflammatory infiltrate.

Management options
Remove the cause of irritation/plaque accumulation (adjust/modify appliance) and scale area thoroughly. Lesions may resolve spontaneously, but if not surgical excision and re-contouring are indicated.

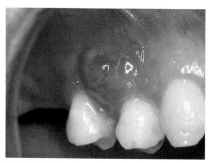

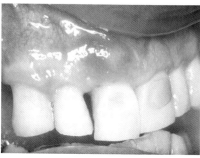

Fig 5-17 A lateral periodontal abscess affecting UR45.

Fig 5-18 A lateral periodontal abscess affecting UR1 - note the colour is creamy rather than the intense red of Fig 5-17.

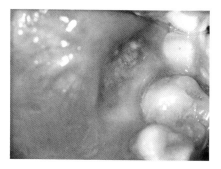

Fig 5-19 A pointing periodontal abscess in the UR6 area.

Lateral Periodontal Abscess

Clinical appearance

This is variable in appearance. It may be a red fluctuant swelling (Fig 5-17) or show evidence of pus beneath (cream appearance, Fig 5-18). It may (Fig 5-19) or may not be 'pointing' and there may be evidence of a sinus tract (Fig 5-20), although most drain via the gingival crevice/periodontal pocket.

Clinical symptoms

Pain/tenderness on lateral pressure usually arises after the gingival swelling has appeared. Pocketing will be evident and there will be a discharge of pus from the pocket or labial sinus tract.

Aetiology

There is microbial infection of the tissues lining the pocket wall, adjacent to an infected root surface. Bacteria are often gram +ve (e.g. Streptococcus constellatus).

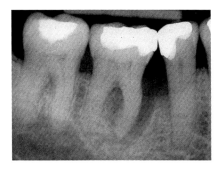
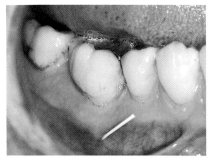

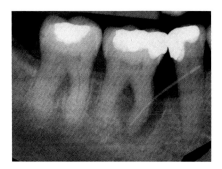

Fig 5-20 A gutta percha point placed within a sinus tract LR5 to trace the source of infection radiographically.

Involvement of non-gingival sites
Patients may rarely become pyrexial, regional lymphadenopathy may be evident and rarely a cellulitis may develop (spreading infection through regional soft tissue planes).

Differential diagnosis
- Giant cell epulis.
- Pyogenic granuloma/vascular epulis.
- Lipoma (if yellow).
- Kaposi's sarcoma (if red).
- Gingival abscess.

Clinical investigation
- Vitality test tooth to eliminate a pulpal aetiology and take periapical radiograph.
- If multiple, consider assessing blood glucose levels.

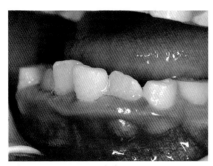 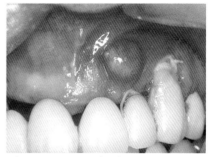

Fig 5-21 A gingival abscess on an erupting LL2 in a child.

Fig 5-22 A stitch abscess UL2 area which has developed superficially around a suture removed five days earlier. This was most likely caused by contaminated suture material being drawn through the tissues during suture removal and following guided tissue regeneration with a non-resorbable membrane UL3.

Management options

Drain the infection directly through the pocket by scaling and root surface debridement (RSD) and curette the pocket wall. If fluctuant, apply topical anaesthesia (e.g. ethyl chloride) and incise with a number 11-scalpel blade. Insert tweezers into cut and open and close to drain pus. If it recurs, consider a swab for culture and sensitivity testing, and if the patient is pyrexial or there is evidence of spreading infection, consider systemic antibiotics.

Gingival Abscess

These are very rare localised purulent infections, usually caused by superficial bacterial infection (e.g. an erupting tooth - Fig 5-21).

Stitch Abscess

Stitch abscesses form beneath soft tissue that has been penetrated by a suture, following a surgical procedure (Fig 5-22). They are rare and normally associated with the use of multi-filament suture materials (e.g. silk). It is believed that the suture becomes colonised by commensal bacteria, some of which track down the suture and beneath the soft tissues, where they cause suppuration and fail to drain. Occasionally, stitch abscesses may also arise after the suture has been removed, due to foreign material being pulled into the tissues as the suture is drawn through. Management involves drainage and if the suture is still present, it should be removed.

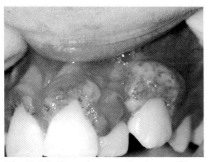 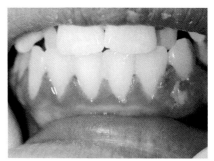

Fig 5-23 Granular exophytic swellings UR1, UL1 and UL3 in a 14-year-old girl who habitually bit her finger nails and irritated her gingivae. She underwent two biopsies before admitting to the habit.

Fig 5-24 Traumatic lesions in the same patient as illustrated in Flig 5-23.

Localised Trauma (see also Chapter 7)

Clinical appearance
Localised chronic gingival trauma can give rise to recession (Chapter 9) if severe, or granular swellings if less aggressive (Fig 5-23 and 5-24). The swellings may be solitary or multiple and appear at the site of the trauma as sessile lesions. There may be superficial ulceration and patches of keratosis and often evidence of granulation tissue formation with a fibrinous surface exudate.

Clinical symptoms
Patients frequently do not complain of pain, although lesions are sore due to the ulceration, and there may be mild surface haemorrhage.

Aetiology
Attention-seeking or habitual scratching with the fingernail or a sharp implement is the most common cause, particularly in teenage females.

Involvement of non-gingival Sites
None.

Differential diagnosis
Lesions can appear sinister if solitary, and differential diagnosis may include:
• Neutropaenia.

99

- Viral warts.
- Squamous cell carcinoma (SCC) of the gingivae.

Clinical investigation
In some cases there should be an incisional biopsy, to exclude an SCC, although this is highly unlikely given the patient's age and lesion location. Histopathology is of non-specific ulceration with chronic inflammation throughout.

Management options
Management needs tact and diplomacy in case there are psychological problems with the child/adolescent or issues surrounding the child–parent relationship. If possible the patient should be approached without parental presence and confirmation of suspicions sought. The patient may on occasion admit to self-abuse, and the discussion alone can encourage habit cessation. Consider the use of chlorhexidine swabs to prevent secondary infection.

Histiocytosis X
Histiocytosis X may present as a localised gingival enlargement, generalised gingival enlargement or indeed as localised recession. The condition is discussed in detail in Chapter 9.

Haemangioma/AV Malformations
Haemangiomas may present as red lesions or gingival swellings and are discussed in Chapter 4.

Kaposi's Sarcoma (KS)
Kaposi's sarcoma is discussed in Chapter 3.

Squamous Cell Carcinoma (SCC)
Squamous cell carcinoma is discussed in Chapter 7, but may present as a localised gingival enlargement.

Metastatic Tumours
Metastatic tumours are rare in the periodontal and gingival tissues. Leukaemic cell infiltration (Chapter 8) may affect the gingiva and metastatic tumours from breast, kidney and prostate do rarely arise. Biopsy is essential for diagnosis.

Lymphoma
Lymphomas are discussed in Chapter 8.

Reactive Osteoma
This is a slow growing benign tumour, which may be reactive to chronic irritation (reactive exostosis) or may appear de novo. It is usually solitary, but multiple lesions may arise as part of Gardner's syndrome a familial autosomal dominant disorder (Chapter 11).

Lesions Associated with PTEN-Hamartoma Tumour Syndromes
(PTEN is a tumour suppressor gene).

Clinical appearance
Benign lesions, largely fibro-epithelial or fibro-vascular in nature may arise on the gingivae, palate, buccal mucosa or tongue. They may appear as:
• Epulides.
• Oral polyps.
• Sessile wart-like lesions.
• Haemangiomatous lesions.

Clinical symptoms
• Swelling.
• Lump that is irritating.
• Incidental finding by patient or GDP.

Aetiology
Germline mutations in the PTEN tumour suppressor gene (PTEN deletions or promoter-region mutations) are associated with two allelic syndromes:
• Cowden's syndrome (90% frequency of PTEN mutations).
• Bannayan-Riley-Ruvalcaba syndrome (BRRS - 65% frequency of PTEN mutations).
• Sub-set of cases of Proteus and Proteus-like syndrome.

Involvement of non-gingival sites
The PTEN gene regulates cell growth, and patients with Cowden's and BRRS syndromes present with multiple hamartomas affecting:
• Lung.
• Breast.
• Skin.
• Glandular tissue (especially thyroid).
• Oral mucosa.
• Polyposis coli.

Haemangiomas and arterio-venous malformations (Chapter 3) are also common.

Differential diagnosis
This may be any common gingival/oral hamartoma or tumour, but patients with Cowden's or BRR syndromes may also have:
• Macrocephaly (large head).
• Learning, speech or organisational difficulties.

Clinical investigation
• Medical history (many cases may be undiagnosed).
• Family history of Cowden's or BRR syndromes.
• Biopsy.

Management options
• Genetic counselling and testing for PTEN mutations.
• Regular recall and fastidious monitoring of the oral mucosa and head and neck are essential.

Footnote
Patients with Cowden's syndrome or BRRS have a frequent need for biopsy and excision of various lesions. Patients are constantly being exposed to medical investigation and minor surgery and require immense support, encouragement and understanding from the dental and medical profession.

Further Reading

Seymour RA, Heasman PH (eds). Drugs Diseases and the Periodontium. Oxford: Oxford Medical Publications, 1992.

Soames JV, Southam JC. (Eds). Oral Pathology. Oxford: Oxford Medical Publications, 1993.

Chapple I L C, Hamburger J. The Significance of Oral Health in HIV Disease. Journal of Sexually Transmitted Infections 2000;76:236-243.

Grattan CEH, Hamburger J. Cowden's disease in two sisters, one showing partial expression. Clinical and Experimental Dermatology 1987;12:360-363.

Chapter 6
Gingival Enlargements – Generalised

Aim

This chapter aims to provide an overview of the causes, features and management of generalised gingival swellings, which involve the free and/or attached gingiva and may also extend to the non-keratinised lining oral mucosa.

Outcome

Having read this chapter, the clinician should be able to formulate an appropriate differential diagnosis for generalised gingival enlargements, know which additional clinical investigations to perform to arrive at a definitive diagnosis and be aware of key management strategies either within their practice or in a specialist environment.

Table 6-1 lists the generalised gingival enlargements discussed in this chapter and highlights which are common and uncommon and when the condition may be managed in general practice or should be referred.

Terminology

A variety of terms has been, and is, used to describe generalised gingival enlargements, which can give rise to confusion. These are summarised below:

Gingival hyperplasia – 'hyperplasia' is a term that describes tissue enlargement arising from an increase in number of one or more constituent cell types. Hyperplasia can therefore be singular (e.g. connective tissue hyperplasia) or compound (e.g. fibro-epithelial hyperplasia). The term gingival hyperplasia has thus become outdated because it poorly describes the true nature of the swelling.

Gingival hypertrophy – 'hypertrophy' describes an increase in tissue size due to an increase in the size of one or more constituent cell types. This can also be singular or compound.

Table 6–1 **Generalised Gingival Swellings**

Appearance/ Character	Category	Sub-Category	Incidence	Manage/ Refer
Fibrous enlargements	Hereditary gingival fibromatosis		uncommon	manage/ refer
	Drug-induced gingival overgrowth	Dilantins (e.g. Phenytoin)	common (13–15% of medicated patients)	manage/ refer
		Calcium channel blocking drugs (e.g. nifedepine amlodipine felodipine)	common (10–15% of medicated patients)	manage/ refer
		Ciclosporin	common (30% of medicated patients)	manage/ refer
	Appliance-induced hyperplasia		common	manage

Appearance/Character	Category	Sub-Category	Incidence	Manage/Refer
	Delayed gingival retreat		common	manage
	Mucopolysaccharidoses		rare	refer
	Mannosidosis		rare	refer
Oedematous enlargements	Inflammatory gingival enlargement	Plaque-induced	common	manage
		Hormonal influence	common	manage
		Hereditary angioedema	uncommon	refer
		Acquired angioedema	uncommon	refer
Granulomatous enlargements	Sarcoidosis		uncommon	refer
	Crohn's Disease		uncommon	refer
	Orofacial Granulomatosis		uncommon	refer
Exophytic swellings	Leukaemia	Acute:		
		monocytic	uncommon	refer
		myelomonocytic	uncommon	refer
		myeloid	uncommon	refer
		lymphocytic	uncommon	refer
	Pyostomatitis vegetans		uncommon	refer
	Wegener's granulomatosis		uncommon	refer
	Plasmacytoma		uncommon	refer
	Amyloidosis		uncommon	refer
	Multiple myeloma		uncommon	refer

Gingival overgrowth – 'overgrowth' is a term used to overcome some of the shortcomings of the above two terms, because it is less specific. The advantage of this term is that it allows for part of, or the entire enlargement to be due to increased production of connective tissue matrix or collagen fibre deposition. 'Overgrowth' is usually used in association with drug-induced enlargements that are histologically complex.

Gingival enlargement – the term 'enlargement' is used in this chapter, because not all gingival enlargements are true swellings (e.g. delayed gingival retreat), but they do appear clinically as enlarged tissues.

Fibrous Swellings

Hereditary Gingival Fibromatosis (HGF)
Clinical appearance
HGF presents as a generalised pink, firm and often stippled enlargement of the free and attached gingivae, extending to the mucogingival junction (see Chapple and Gilbert, 2002) buccally extending variably into the palate. Classically it affects maxillary tuberosities (Fig 6-1) and retromolar regions of the mandible (Fig 6-2). However, the labial gingivae may be involved (Fig 6-3), and it is important to distinguish this from delayed gingival retreat if planning surgical recontouring. The fibrosis is slowly progressive and may give rise to tooth movement and spacing, or may delay or prevent tooth eruption.

Clinical symptoms
The patient's main concerns will be:
• Aesthetic.
• Functional – tissue can overgrow the crowns of teeth if severe. Also teeth may be moved to a position that interferes with normal occlusal function.
• Discomfort – can arise where fibrosis is actively moving teeth.

Aetiology
Unknown, but two forms are described:
• Familial HGF – autosomal dominant inheritance recently linked (Hart et al, 1998) to chromosome 2p21 (position 21 of short arm of chromosome 2). Penetrance may be incomplete, i.e. the condition may not always be expressed phenotypically or may vary in severity.
• Sporadic HGF – a controversial diagnosis that may be autosomal dominant or recessive. It may simply be a familial form that has variable clini-

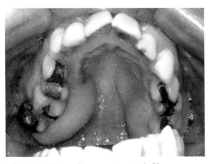

Fig 6-1 Hereditary gingival fibromatosis classically affecting the maxillary tuberosities, where false pocketing had led to early periodontal attachment loss.

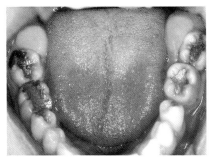

Fig 6-2 Hereditary gingival fibromatosis classically affecting the mandibular retromolar region.

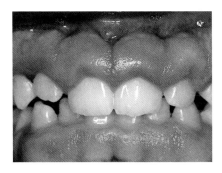

Fig 6-3 Hereditary gingivo-fibromatosis of the labial gingivae in a 12-year- old boy, whose mother, aunt and younger brother were also affected.

cal expression, incomplete penetrance or may arise due to a spontaneous mutation within the 2p21 region.

Involvement of non-gingival sites
Gingival fibromatosis is also associated with various rare syndromes:

- Rutherford syndrome (juvenile hyaline fibrosis, corneal dystrophy, neurosensory hearing loss) – autosomal dominant inheritance.
- Laband syndrome (nail, ear, nose and bone defects, syndactyly) – autosomal recessive/dominant or spontaneous mutations.
- Cross syndrome (hypopigmentation, microphthalmia, athetosis) – autosomal recessive.
- Ramon syndrome (hypertrichosis [excessive hair growth], cherubism, mental retardation) – autosomal recessive.

Hypertrichosis, mental retardation, epilepsy and growth hormone defects are also described by Gorlin et al (1976), and interestingly hypertrichosis and

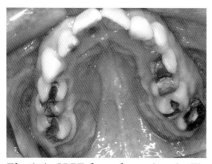

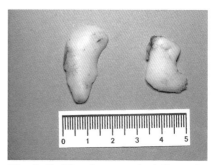

Fig 6-4a HGF from the patient in Fig 6-1, immediately post–open-face gingivectomy.

Fig 6-4b The tissue excised from the patient in Fig 6-4a.

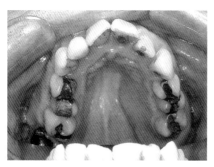

Fig 6-5 The healed tuberosities from 6-4a, two weeks post-surgery. False pocketing has been eliminated. Note the improved angle between the gingival margin UL6 and the tooth, facilitating ease of plaque control.

gingival fibrosis are both complications of ciclosporin medication (see below).

Differential diagnosis
- Delayed gingival retreat.
- Drug-induced gingival overgrowth.
- Plaque-induced chronic inflammatory enlargement.

Clinical investigation
HGF is a presumptive diagnosis based on a careful history and clinical findings. Definitive diagnosis currently requires confirmatory histopathology in addition to clinical findings. Excision biopsy is usually by conventional open-faced gingivectomy (Fig 6-4, 6-5), but if severe, an inverse bevel flap may be required (Fig 6-6) with significant undermining by sharp dissection and filleting ± a distal wedge procedure (Fig 6-7).

Fig 6-6 Diagram to illustrate the inverse bevel incision prior to flap reflection and 'filleting' of the bulk of the sub-mucosal connective tissue.

a. Bulky tissue prior to split-thickness flap reflection.
b. First incision is parallel to a sulcus incision, using an inverse bevel.
c. Second incision isolates a tissue 'cuff'.
d. Split-thickness flap is then raised by sharp dissection allowing surgical access to the underside of the flap.
e. Cuff is removed and underside of flap is debulked by sharp excision of excess connective tissue. Care must be taken to avoid puncturing the flap.
f. Flap is closed after any necessary debridement and removal of the bulky connective tissue from the underside of the flap.

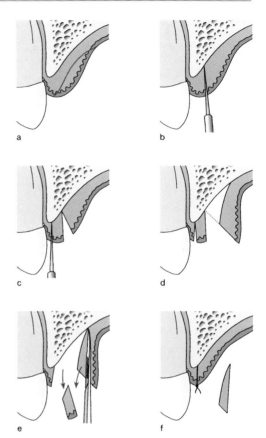

Management

If mild and symptom-free, simply monitor. However, probing is essential to distinguish between true and false pocketing (Fig 6-8). Surgical reduction is likely to require specialist skills for tuberosity and retromolar lesions, as feeder arteries can arise within, and the sublingual space may be compromised during lower molar surgery. Slow recurrence is likely.

Drug-induced Gingival Overgrowth (DIGO)
Clinical appearance

The appearance of DIGO is variable. Classically the enlargement starts at the interdental papilla and spreads to involve the marginal gingivae. The ante-

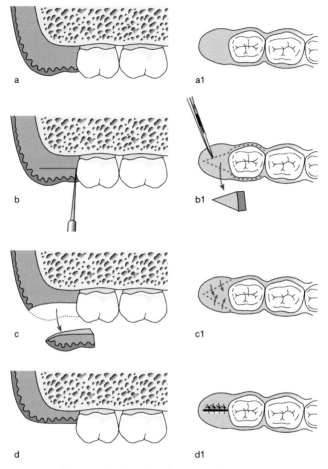

Fig 6-7 Diagram to illustrate the distal wedge procedure. There are several variants, but the most basic literally involves the sharp dissection of a wedge of tissue from the tuberosity/retro-molar region.

a.   Enlarged tuberosity with false pocketing distal to UR7.

a1. Occlusal view of 'a'.

b.   A buccal and lingual/palatal incision is made down to the alveolar crest

b1. The wedge is delineated by the dotted lines and buccal and palatal flaps are raised a short distance prior to wedge removal.

c.   Wedge is sharp-dissected out.

c1. Buccal and lingual flaps are approximated over 'dead space' and in doing so this space is eliminated and the tissue level falls.

d.   View of closed defect with tissue level more apically positioned.

d1. Occlusal view with distal wedge removal complete and flaps sutured.

110

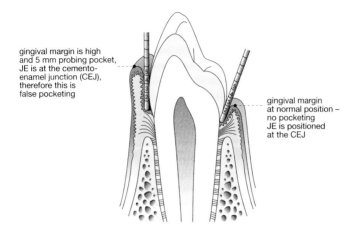

Fig 6-8 Schematic longitudinal section of a premolar and associated periodontal tissues demonstrating a healthy sulcus and false pocketing.

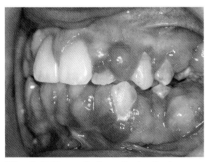

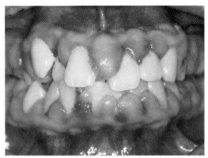

Fig 6-9 Drug-induced gingival overgrowth in a renal transplant patient medicated with ciclosporin. Molar teeth were covered making mastication uncomfortable.

Fig 6-10 Fibrous overgrowth in a patient medicated with ciclosporin.

rior gingivae are most commonly affected, but posterior enlargement may lead to occlusal surface coverage in severe cases (Fig 6-9). With phenytoin and ciclosporin, in the presence of good plaque control, overgrowth is firm, fibrous and pink (Fig 6-10), but where plaque control is poor it becomes more vascular (Fig 6-11). Overgrowth associated with calcium channel blocking drugs (CCBs) tends to be more vascular (Fig 6-12) and is associated with more severe enlargement with concurrent ciclosporin. Surface keratosis or ulceration may arise following trauma from opposing teeth.

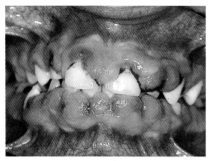

Fig 6-11 DIGO with a more vascular inflammatory component due to poor plaque control. (Fig 7-5 book 11).

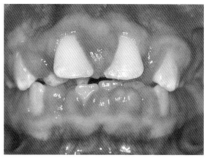

Fig 6-12 Fibro-vascular overgrowth in a patient medicated with ciclosporin and nifedepine.

Clinical symptoms
As for HGF.

Aetiology
DIGO is associated classically with three drug types, but has also been reported with the oral contraceptive, cannabis (Rees, 1992), erythromycin (Valsecchi and Cainelli, 1992) and sodium valproate (Syrjanen & Sryjanen 1979).
- Calcium channel blocking (CCB) drugs – nifedepine, amlodipine, felodipine, diltiazem hydrochloride.
- Dilantins – phenytoin
- Ciclosporin.

CCBs are used to control hypertension, ciclosporin is an immunosuppressive agent used to modulate allograft rejection or in severe erosive mucosal disease (Chapter 8). Phenytoin is an anti-convulsant drug. While there are some common features to their modes of action at an ionic level, the aetiology of DIGO remains poorly understood and complex. Seymour et al (2000) have described a number of risk factors:

• Age		+ve
• Genetic	– HLA-DR2 for Ciclosporin	+ve
	– HLA-B37 for Ciclosporin	–ve
• Gender	– Male	+ve
	– Female	–ve
• Periodontal variables	– Gingival inflammation	+++ve
	– Plaque	++ve

- Concomitant   - Ciclosporin and CCBs   +++ve
  medication   - Phenytoin and hepatic enzyme inducers   +ve
                - Ciclosporin and azathioprine   –ve
                - Ciclosporin and prednisolone   –ve
- Drug   - Pre-transplant enlargement   +ve
  variables   - Plasma concentrations   +ve
                - Gingival crevicular fluid (GCF) concentrations   +ve
                - Salivary concentration   +ve

Involvement of non-gingival sites
There are isolated reports of DIGO arising on an edentulous ridge. Hypertrichosis is associated with DIGO during ciclosporin medication.

Differential diagnosis
- HGF.
- Delayed gingival retreat.
- Plaque-induced chronic inflammatory overgrowth.
- Pyostomatitis vegetans.
- Leukaemia.
- C1-esterase inhibitor deficiency (Hereditary angioedema) – Roberts et al, 2003.

Clinical investigation
Diagnosis is made following a careful drug history and clinical examination (Chapter 1). Excisional biopsy demonstrates a fibroepithelial hyperplasia with epithelial acanthosis and increases in fibroblast number and/or collagen and extracellular matrix production. There is some evidence from immuno-histochemistry for the involvement of growth factors such as transforming growth factor beta (TGFβ: Wright et al, 2001).

Management
A staged approach is necessary:
1. Hygiene-phase therapy (OHI and scaling) to reduce the inflammatory component.
2. Liaise with medical specialist to change medication if appropriate – spontaneous resolution with time (months) often results.
   - for ciclosporin, replacement with tacrolimus (FK-506) may be justified to prevent the need for repeat surgery in severe and recurrent cases.
   - for CCBs it may be possible to replace with a β-blocker, ACE-inhibitor or diuretic, or a combination of these.

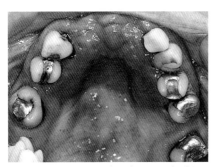 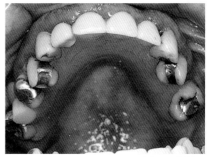

Fig 6-13a An acrylic denture lacking tooth support.

Fig 6-13b Denture stomatitis and false pocketing UL 234 as a result of the poorly designed prosthesis in Fig 6-13a.

- where CCBs are in concomitant use with ciclosporin, CCB replacement initially is the best approach.
3. If swelling remains a problem, surgical gingival recontouring.
4. Rigorous supportive care (see Heasman, Preshaw and Robertson, 2004).

For subjects who have had a renal transplant ± chronic end-stage renal failure, calcium metabolism is disrupted and hypercalcaemia results in cardiac valve calcification in up to 50% of cases (Ribeiro et al, 1998). Antimicrobial prophylaxis will therefore be needed. Renal transplant patients who have an arterio-venous fistula from haemodialysis, and foreign bodies in their vasculature to support the shunt, may also require such prophylaxis. For heart, lung, liver transplants and prosthetic joint replacements, there is no current evidence to support the use of antibiotic cover.

Dental Appliance-induced Enlargement
Clinical appearance
The appearance of appliance-induced enlargement is of thickened and enlarged (normally palatal) gingival tissues arising beneath a poorly designed prosthetic appliance base (Fig 6-13). Such appliances are tissue-borne and give rise to false pocketing (Fig 6-4) secondary to coronal up-growth of the gingiva. The tissues can become inflamed with time and a thin, red mobile margin develops.

Clinical symptoms
Occasionally an unstable prosthesis or discomfort and bleeding on brushing.

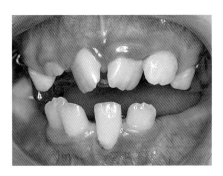

Fig 6-14 Delayed gingival retreat. The gingival margins around all upper incisors and three of the four lower incisors have not reached their mature 'adult' position. The margin at LL1 is prematurely at its adult position and may progress to recession.

Aetiology
Lesions directly related to irritation by appliance components are caused by a chronic inflammatory reaction, leading to fibrovascular hyperplasia.

Involvement of non-gingival sites
None.

Differential diagnosis
The diagnosis is usually obvious following examination of the prosthesis in situ.

Clinical investigation
Excisional biopsy shows fibroepithelial hyperplasia with a chronic inflammatory infiltrate.

Management options
Adjust/modify the appliance initially and scale area thoroughly. Surgical excision is likely to be needed, but lesions rarely resolve spontaneously. Re-make a definitive prosthesis that eliminates the original design flaw (see Noble, Kellett and Chapple, 2004).

Delayed Gingival Retreat
Clinical appearance
Short clinical crowns, give the impression that the free and attached gingivae have overgrown (Fig 6-14). The attached gingivae are not thickened, but there may be rolling of the free gingival margin and mild thickening.

Clinical symptoms
Patients include children, adolescents or young adults (see Clerehugh, Tugnait and Chapple, 2004), who may complain of a 'gummy smile' or that their peer group make fun of them because they 'have no teeth'.

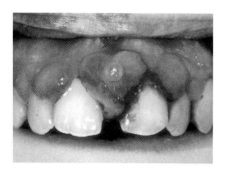

Fig 6-15 Inflammatory gingival enlargement, due to plaque accumulation aggravated by pregnancy in a young patient.

Aetiology
Biologically slow retreat of the gingival margin to its mature adult position, 2-3mm coronal to the cemento-enamel junction (CEJ).

Involvement of non-gingival sites
None.

Differential diagnosis
• HGF.
• DIGO.
• Variation in normal anatomy (see Chapple and Gilbert, 2002).

Clinical investigation
Clinical examination alone.

Management options
• Check for true pocketing.
• Reassure patients and parents and review the situation after 12 months.

Oedematous Enlargements

Inflammatory Gingival Enlargement
Clinical appearance
Red, swollen marginal gingivae with a degree of fibrosis (Fig 6-15). False pocketing results from coronal overgrowth and with time may lead to true pocketing.

Clinical symptoms
Bleeding on brushing, soreness, malodour and aesthetic concerns.

116

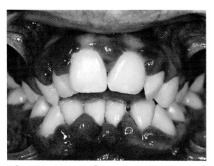

Fig 6-16 Inflammatory gingival enlargement, due to plaque accumulation aggravated by a reduced ability to clean around imbricated teeth.

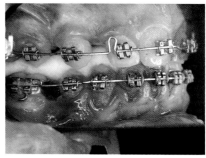

Fig 6-17 Mild inflammatory gingival enlargement, due to plaque accumulation aggravated by the presence of a fixed orthodontic appliance.

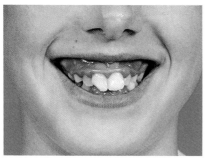

Fig 6-18a A 12-year-old boy who breathes through his mouth, with a high lip line and incompetent lips.

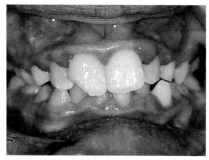

Fig 6-18b Mild inflammatory gingival enlargement in 12-year-old boy who breathes through his mouth with a high lip line and incompetent lips. A lack of saliva flow also reduces cleansing and aggravates the situation.

Aetiology
Poor plaque control initially leads to plaque-induced gingivitis. If unresolved, the inflammatory lesion becomes chronic and fibrous repair occurs concurrently with plaque-induced inflammation. Generally the enlargement or 'hyperplastic response' arises due to the presence of local risk factors that inhibit plaque removal and directly irritate the tissues. These include:
- Imbricated teeth (Fig 6-16).
- Orthodontic appliances (Fig 6-17).
- Mouth breathing (Fig 6-18).

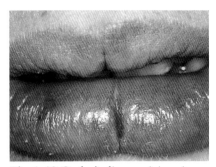

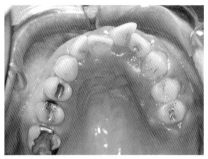

Fig 6-19 Crohn's disease giving rise to a midline lip fissure due to the marked oedema. Angioedema presents in a similar manner, but without the midline fissuring.

Fig 6-20 Severe gingival oedema in a patient who has C1-esterase inhibitor deficiency (hereditary angioedema type II).

- Hormonal – puberty or pregnancy result in hormonal changes and the gingival and periodontal tissues possess oestradiol and androgen receptors. The latter appear to induce histological changes which include epithelial separation and increases in vascular permeability (Vittek et al, 1984; Jönsson et al, 2004). Gingival tissues are also capable of sex steroid metabolism (El Attar, 1974), and the inflammatory response to plaque accumulation may be exaggerated at such stages in life.

Histology shows collagen fibres, fibroblasts and inflammatory cells.

Involvement of non-gingival sites
None.

Differential diagnosis
- Appliance-induced enlargement.
- DIGO.

Clinical investigation
Additional investigations are not indicated, given the presence of plaque deposits and associated risk factors.

Management options
Treatment should include scaling and oral hygiene instruction in the first instance, with regular supportive care. This will resolve the inflammatory component of the enlargement, but any remaining fibrous deformity should be corrected surgically.

Angioedema (C1-Esterase Inhibitor Deficiency/Dysfunction)
Angioedema may be caused by a C1-esterase inhibitor defect or, indeed, may have an allergic aetiology. The discussion in this section will not cover the allergic form.

Clinical appearance
Angioedema classically presents with lip swelling (Fig 6-19) or angioedema of the head, neck or extremities. Onset is acute. Extremely rarely, gingival tissues may be involved (Fig 6-20) in an obscure localised form of angioedema (Roberts et al, 2003).

Clinical symptoms
Aesthetics, discomfort and concern over the swelling are the main reasons for presentation. Additionally, oedema of the tongue, cheeks and upper and lower airways often leads to dyspnoea (breathlessness), which can, in severe cases, be life threatening.

Aetiology
Angioedema may be hereditary (HAO) or acquired (allergic) in nature. It involves a defect in an enzyme that damps down complement activation (see Chapple and Gilbert 2002). The acquired form usually presents in adults but HAO, which has an autosomal dominant pattern of inheritance, can present in younger patients.

HAO is classified into:
• Type I HAO – a decrease in production of enzyme.
• Type II HAO – normal enzyme levels but dysfunctional enzyme.

Involvement of non-gingival sites
• Tongue.
• Cheeks.
• Upper airway.
• Head.
• Neck.
• Extremities.

Differential diagnosis
• Oro-facial granulomatosis (OFG).
• Crohn's disease.
• Sarcoidosis.
• Type I hypersensitivity reaction.

Clinical investigation
Assay levels of C1, C1-esterase inhibitor and also C1-esterase inhibitor function in plasma.

Management options
Medical management is complex and may involve intravenous administration of C1-esterase inhibitor concentrate, or use of anabolic steroids such as stanozolol or danazol. Referral to a clinical immunologist is essential.

Granulomatous Enlargements

Orofacial Granulomatosis (OFG)
OFG is not a diagnosis, more a descriptive term that reflects underlying disease, such as:
• Hypersensitivity reactions to dietary allergens.
• Sarcoidosis.
• Angioedema.
• Melkersson-Rosenthal syndrome.
• Crohn's Disease.
• TB.
• Leprosy.

Clinical appearance
The clinical appearance and symptoms of OFG are essentially those of 'oral Crohn's disease' (see above), but the gastrointestinal features are absent. It usually presents in the second or third decade of life and has an equal sex ratio.

Aetiology
The aetiology of OFG is obscure, and the term is often used to describe oral granulomatous conditions with no known systemic cause. There is evidence that OFG may be due to hypersensitivity reactions to dietary allergens such as benzoates and cinnamonaldehyde.

Involvement of non-gingival sites
• Facial/lip swelling.
• Mucosal ulceration.
• Mucosal tags and cobblestoning.
• Extra-oral involvement.

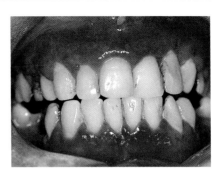

Fig 6-21 A broad 'band-like' gingival erythema with a soft 'velvet-like' consistency. Biopsy and subsequent investigations confirmed sarcoidosis.

Clinical investigation
- Biopsy down to muscle is needed and shows non-caseating epithelioid cell granulomata and lymphoedema.
- Blood investigations may indicate raised serum ACE (angiotensin-converting enzyme) levels, due to ACE release from the granulomas.
- Chest radiographs.

Management options
- The underlying cause if identified, should be treated, but this may not affect resolution of orofacial swelling. If allergens are identified by skin testing, these should be avoided through employment of exclusion diets.
- Intralesional corticosteroids may provide short-term relief, as may surgical reduction.

Sarcoidosis
Clinical appearance
- Broad-band granular gingival erythema (Fig 6-21).
- Velvet-like consistency to free and attached gingivae.
- Gingival swelling may extend beyond mucogingival junction.
- Lip swelling may occur.
- Cervical lymphadenopathy.
- Salivary gland enlargement is rarely associated with Heerfordt's syndrome, which includes a facial palsy, lacrimal swelling, uveitis and fever.

Clinical symptoms
- Discomfort is described in some patients.
- Aesthetic concerns.

Aetiology
Sarcoidosis is a rare (0.02% in Caucasians) multifocal granulomatous disorder, more common in black patients.

Involvement of non-gingival sites
- Lungs.
- Spleen.
- Liver.
- Eyes.
- Salivary (parotid) glands (Heerfordt's syndrome).
- Skin.
- Lymph nodes – hilar (lung) and cervical.

Differential diagnosis
- Crohn's Disease.
- Melkersson-Rosenthal syndrome (facial oedema/swelling, plicated tongue and a VII nerve palsy).

Clinical investigation
- Biopsy may aid diagnosis, identifying non-caseating giant cell granulomas.
- Chest radiograph may show lung involvement.
- Blood tests for angiotensin converting enzyme (ACE), which can be raised in serum due to its production by the tissue granulomas.

Management options
Refer to a physician. Medical management involves treatment with systemic corticosteroids and has a high success rate.

Crohn's Disease
Crohn's disease is a chronic inflammatory granulomatous bowel disease. It typically affects the ileum or colon, but may affect any part of the digestive system. The affected areas become red and swollen and ulceration may arise. As the ulcers heal, scar tissue forms, inducing intestinal strictures and obstruction.

Clinical appearance
- Broad-band gingival swelling.
- Mucosal tags.
- Linear 'fissured' ulceration of oral mucosa.
- Cobblestone appearance to the buccal mucosa due to fibrosis of ulcers.
- Lip swelling with a linear midline fissure (Fig 6-19).

Clinical symptoms
- Swollen gingivae/lips.
- Oral ulceration.
- Cracking of corners of mouth (angular stomatitis).

Aetiology
Crohn's is a chronic inflammatory bowel disease of unknown aetiology.

Involvement of non-gingival sites
- Small bowel, patients may pass blood and mucous per rectum with loose stools/diarrhoea.

Differential diagnosis
- OFG.
- Sarcoidosis.
- Melkersson-Rosenthal syndrome.
- Angioedema.

Clinical investigation
- Biopsy is needed for diagnosis, where granulomas and lymphoedema are characteristic.
- Blood tests may reveal low serum iron, B12 due to malabsorption.
- Gastrointestinal investigation of the terminal ileum by barium imaging.

Management options
Medical management requires specialist referal to gastroenterology. Oral management is often unsatisfactory and may involve the use of topical corticosteroid preparations or intralesional corticosteroid injections (triamcinolone). Specialist referal is required.

Exophytic Swellings

Leukaemia
Leukaemia may present as generalised gingival enlargement, but also as ulceration or haemorrhage (see Chapter 8).

Pyostomatitis Vegetans
Clinical appearance
- Irregular gingival swelling appearing somewhat granular and warty.
- Yellow pustular appearance due to intra/sub-epithelial abscesses.
- Areas of necrosis and sloughing.

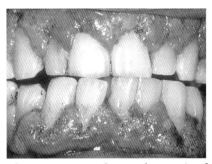

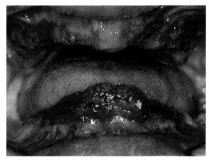

Fig 6-22 Wegener's granulomatosis of gingivae.

Fig 6-23 Wegener's granulomatosis in an adult, presenting as a strawberry-like granular swelling of the lower alveolus.

- Exophytic appearance.
- Profuse bleeding.

Clinical symptoms
- Swollen gums.
- Gingivae are sore/painful.
- Bleeding gums.
- Malodour.
- Aesthetic concerns over appearance.
- May have gastrointestinal symptomatology.

Aetiology
Extremely rare and is associated with inflammatory bowel disease (occasionally Crohn's, but more usually ulcerative colitis). The patient in Fig 1-7 presented with triple pathology: NUG, erosive lichen planus and pyostomatitis vegetans.

Involvement of non-gingival sites
- Labial/buccal mucosa.
- Alveolar mucosa.

Differential diagnosis
- Acute leukaemia.
- DIGO with severe inflammation and ulceration from trauma.
- Vesiculobullous disease.
- Wegener's granulomatosis.

Clinical investigation
- Consider serological and haematological investigations to identify possible malabsoption (e.g. iron and vit B12) and elevation of acute phase markers.
- Biopsy to demonstrate tissue abscess formation.
- Endoscopy.

Management options
Management is medical and involves controlling underlying bowel disease. Reduce any sources of oral infection (extract teeth with poor prognosis) and treat any associated periodontal disease.

Wegener's Granulomatosis
Clinical appearance
- Granular 'strawberry-like' gingival hyperplasia (Fig 6-22).
- Exophytic strawberry-like lesions may develop (Fig 6-23).
- Delayed healing of extraction sockets.

Clinical symptoms
- Swollen gums.
- Gingivae can be painful and ulceration is described.
- Chronic sinusitis or nasal obstruction.

Aetiology
Systemic disease of unknown aetiology, but an immunological basis is suspected.

Involvement of non-gingival sites
- Classically necrotising granulomas of the nose, paranasal sinuses and lungs.
- Small artery vasculitis of respiratory tract and lungs.
- Renal vasculitis (glomerulitis).
- Tongue may be involved.

Differential diagnosis
- DIGO
- Pyostomatitis vegetans.

Clinical investigation
- Biopsy shows necrotising vascular changes in small vessels, granulation tissue, microabscess formation and non-specific inflammation involving most forms of leukocyte within tissues (histiocytes). There may be an epithelial hyperplasia and giant cells are common.

- Blood investigations show anti-neutrophil cytoplasmic antibodies (ANCA) in serum (cytoplasmic staining with specificity for proteinase 3).

Management options
- Urgent referral to appropriate medical specialty (renal medicine or rheumatology):
  - Medical management may involve the use of systemic corticosteroids (prednisolone) or cytotoxics (cyclophosphamide).
  - Monitoring of serum ANCA levels, which vary with disease activity.

Bony Swellings

These are discussed in Chapter 11.

Further Reading

Chapple ILC, Gilbert AD. Understanding Periodontal Diseases: Assessment and Diagnostic Procedures and Practice. Chapple ILC (ed). QuintEssentials of Dental Practice −1, Periodontology-1. London: Quintessence Publishing Co. Ltd, 2002;Chapter 1,pp3-16.

Clerehugh V, Tugnait A, Chapple ILC. Periodontal Management of Children, Adolescents and Young Adults. 2004. Chapple ILC (ed). QuintEssentials of Dental Practice −17, Periodontology-4. London: Quintessence Publishing Co. Ltd, 2004;Chapter 10,pp131-149.

Gorlin RJ, Pindborg JJ, Cohen MM Jr. (Eds). Syndromes of the Head and Neck. 2nd Edn. New York: McGraw-Hill, 1976;pp329-336.

El Attar TMA. The in vitro conversion of male sex steroid 1,2-3H-androstenedione in normal and inflamed human gingivae. Arch Oral Biol 1974;19:1185-1190.

Heasman PA, Preshaw PM, Robertson P. Successful Periodontal Therapy. A Non-Surgical Approach. Chapple ILC (ed). QuintEssentials of Dental Practice −16, Periodontology-3. London: Quintessence Publishing Co. Ltd, 2004;Chapter 9 pp99-133.

Jönsson D, Andersson G, Ekblad E, Liang M, Bratthall G, Nilsson B-O. Imunocytochemical demonstration of oestrogen , in human periodontal ligament cells. Archives of Oral Biology 2004;49:85-88.

Noble SN, Kellett M, Chapple ILC. Decision Making for the Periodontal Team. Chapple ILC (Ed). QuintEssentials of Dental Practice −11, Periodontology-2, London: Quintessence Publishing Co. Ltd, 2004;Chapter 10 pp131-149.

Rees TD. Oral effects of drug abuse. Crit Rev Oral Biol Med 1992;3:163-184.

Ribeiro S, Ramos A, Brandao et al. Cardiac valve calcification in haemodialysis patients: role of calcium-phosphate metabolism. Nephrol Dial Transplant 1998;13:2037-2040.

Roberts A, Shah M, Chapple ILC. C-1 esterase inhibitor dysfunction localised to the periodontal tissues: clues to the role of stress in the pathogenesis of chronic periodontitis? J Clin Periodontol 2003;30:271-277.

Seymour RA, Heasman PH (eds). Drugs Diseases and the Periodontium. Oxford: Oxford Medical Publications, 1992.

Seymour RA, Ellis JS, Thomason JM. Risk factors for drug-induced gingival overgrowth. J Clin Periodontol 2000;27:217-223.

Vittek J, Kirsch S, Rappaport SC, Bergman M, Southren AL. Salivary concentrations of steroid hormones in males and in cycling and post-menopausal females with and without periodontitis. J Perio Res 1984;19:545-555.

Wright HJ, Chapple ILC, Matthews JB. TGF, isoforms and receptors in drug-induced and hereditary gingival overgrowth. J Oral Pathol Med 2001;30:281-289.

Chapter 7
Localised Gingival Ulceration

Aim

The aim of this chapter is to detail those clinical entities that may present as a single or isolated discrete area of ulceration on the gingiva, as opposed to more widespread or multiple areas of ulceration.

Outcome

The reader should be able to differentiate between the sinister and the trivial, request relevant investigations and appropriately manage the conditions discussed.

Definition

Gingival ulceration describes an area of mucosa devoid of its surface epithelium, and exposing the underlying connective tissue.

The term 'erosion' is sometimes used to describe those areas of shallow ulceration that do not expose the underlying connective tissue. Table 7-1 provides a summary of the contents of this chapter.

Traumatic Ulceration
Traumatic ulceration of the gingiva has a variety of causes including:
- Iatrogenic, (ill-fitting or ill-designed oral appliances and inappropriate oral hygiene practices).
- Self-induced (gingivitis artefacta) - (Fig 7-1) see Chapter 9.
- Direct chemical toxicity (dentifrices, aspirin or the use of recreational drugs such as cocaine) - see Chapters 3 and 10.

Clinical appearance
- Traumatic ulceration varies in appearance dependent on the causative factors. The site of ulceration may identify the source of the trauma, for example a clasp on a denture, a spring on an orthodontic appliance or malpositioned teeth.

Table 7-1 **Summary table – localised gingival ulceration**

Major Categories	Sub Categories	Frequency of Condition	Management Setting
Trauma	Iatrogenic (from dental appliances) Chemical / Thermal Gingivitis artefacta	Traumatic ulceration of the gingivae occurs frequently.	These conditions can usually be managed by non-specialists although if psychiatric morbidity is associated with gingivitis artefacta, appropriate referral is necessary.
Recurrent aphthous stomatitis	Minor aphthous ulceration Major aphthous ulceration Herpetiform aphthous ulceration	Aphthous stomatitis is a very common condition (reportedly affecting 20% of the UK population).	Gingival involvement is however unusual. Initial management is undertaken in primary care. If there is a suggestion of underlying disease or poor response to treatment, the patient should be referred for a specialist opinion.
Neoplasia	Usually squamous cell carcinoma Lymphomas Leukaemias Metastatic tumours Benign tumours	Oral mucosal neoplasia is uncommon and gingival involvement is rare.	Urgent referral for specialist management of malignancy.

Major Categories	Sub Categories	Frequency of Condition	Management Setting
Bacterial infections	Necrotising ulcerative gingivitis	Uncommon	Manage in primary care Refer if patient's immune status is suspect.
	Tuberculosis	Very rare	
	Syphilis	Very rare	Specialist referral
Viral infections	Hand, foot and mouth	Uncommon	Supportive management within primary care setting
	Varicella zoster	Uncommonly affects the gingivae	Primary care or referral dependent on distribution and severity
	Cytomegalovirus	Very rare	Referral – condition indicative of compromised immunity
Deep mycoses	Histoplasmosis	Very rare in the UK	Specialist referral

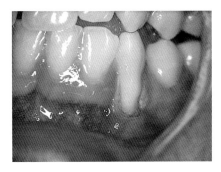

Fig 7-1 Gingivitis artefacta.

- The appearance is one of non-specific ulceration that may mirror very closely the source of the trauma.
- Self-induced trauma can have dramatic clinical consequences including exfoliation of the teeth.

Clinical symptoms
- Patients may be asymptomatic but are more likely to complain of soreness at the area of the ulceration.
- In gingivitis artefacta the patient may well be a young adult or adolescent.

Involvement of non-gingival sites
- Localised ulceration of the gingivae is not usually associated with extragingival involvement although direct chemical toxicity and physical trauma from dental prostheses or orthodontic appliances may also provoke similar manifestations on the oral mucosa.
- Patients who self-harm may also traumatise themselves elsewhere.

Differential diagnosis
- Non-specific ulceration.
- Vesiculobullous disease.
- Tumours.
- Wegener's granulomatosis.
- Pyostomatitis vegetans.
- Stewart's midline granuloma.

Clinical investigation
- Clinical history and examination is essential and will reveal obvious local sources of trauma.
- Assessment of the psychological demeanour of the patient is paramount

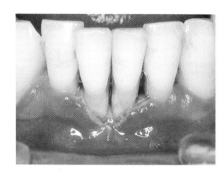

Fig 7-2 Ulceration of the interdental papillae in necrotising ulcerative gingivitis.

when self-harm is suspected. Direct questioning may well not elicit a truthful response, patients often strongly denying such activity.
• Biopsy of lesions is useful to exclude other diagnoses.

Management options
• Elimination of obvious sources of trauma.
• In cases of self-harm, urgent referral for psychiatric advice is appropriate.
• In cases of suspected self-harm where there is significant injury, admission to hospital for supervision may be necessary to establish a definitive diagnosis.

Bacterial Infections

Bacterial infections producing discrete localised areas of ulceration of the gingivae are uncommon.

Necrotising Ulcerative Gingivitis (NUG)
See also Chapter 9, Localised Gingival Recession.

Clinical appearance
• Ragged ulceration and necrosis involving the interdental papillae (Fig 7-2).
• Lesional tissue covered by a fibrinopurulent grey slough.
• Gingival bleeding and inflammation.

Clinical symptoms
• The lesions are painful.
• Characteristic foetor oris (bad breath).
• Bad taste in mouth.

Aetiology
- Anaerobic infection with a variety of organisms including Treponema vincentii and Fusobacterium nucleatum constituting the so called 'fusospirachaetal complex'. In addition Prevotella intermedia is also reported to be associated with NUG. The risk factors that predispose to NUG include:
  - Poor oral hygiene.
  - Smoking.
  - Immunodeficiency.
  - Malnutrition.
  - Concurrent infections.

Involvement of non-gingival sites
- The infection can extend to adjacent tissues, including other periodontal tissues and the oral mucosa.
- In severe cases, in the debilitated or immunocompromised, the condition may involve the skin and can be extremely destructive (cancrum oris).

Differential diagnosis
- Myeloproliferative disease.
- Immunocompromised host.

Clinical investigation
- The diagnosis is usually made on the clinical features.
- Laboratory identification of the fusospirochaetal complex.

Management options
- Oral hygiene instruction.
- Smoking cessation.
- Scaling and root surface debridement.
- Correction of underlying predisposing factors such as malnutrition.
- Oral metronidazole 200-400mg three times daily for three days.

Tuberculosis
Although cases of tuberculosis are increasing in incidence, oral and particularly gingival manifestations remain infrequent.

The infection may manifest on the gingivae as a solitary ulcer with irregular and often undermined margins. It may also be painless and usually results from secondary infection due to expectorated infected sputum.

Syphilis

The prevalence of sexually transmitted infections has increased dramatically over the last decade. Reported cases of syphilis in the UK are now at their highest level since 1984, with a six-fold rise in males occurring since 1998.

The primary site of infection with Treponema pallidum produces the so-called 'chancre' – this occurs at a variable time after inoculation, but usually of the order of three weeks later. The initial lesion is of a papule that ulcerates. The resultant chancre is indurated, often painless, associated with regional lymphadenopathy and resolves spontaneously within two to three weeks. (Alam, 2000). Gingival involvement is rare, intra-oral lesions being more frequently seen on the lips, tongue and palatal mucosa.

The superficial erosions or mucous patches ('snail track ulcers') of secondary syphilis are a rare gingival finding although intra-oral lesions may occur in up to 40% of cases, typically arising some four to ten weeks after the chancre. The gumma of tertiary syphilis has not been reported to involve the gingivae.

Diagnostic confirmation depends on serological testing and histological examination of the lesion may also be undertaken to exclude other diagnoses.

Viral Infections

Viral infections, such as primary herpes simplex, often produce generalised gingival or oral mucosal involvement (see Chapter 4). However the following infections may produce more limited gingival involvement.

Hand, Foot and Mouth Disease
Clinical appearance
- Small vesicles that rupture to produce superficial ulcerations that coalesce forming serpiginous areas reminiscent of herpes simplex infection (Fig 7-3, 7-4).
- There is no inflammatory gingivitis as may be seen in primary herpes infections, although the ulcers are surrounded by an inflammatory halo.

Clinical symptoms
- The infection is usually mild with little systemic upset, limiting itself in 10–14 days.
- Soreness at the site of the ulceration.

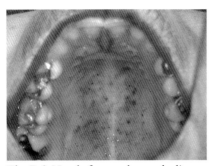 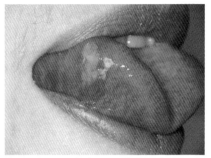

Fig 7-3 Hand, foot and mouth disease involving the palatal mucosa.

Fig 7-4 Hand, foot and mouth disease showing coalescence of burst vesicles on the tongue.

Aetiology
- Infection is usually with Coxsackie A16.

Involvement of non-gingival sites
- Any intra–oral site may be affected.
- Palms of the hands, soles of the feet and other areas of the skin subject to minor trauma.

Differential diagnosis
- Herpes simplex infection.
- Erythema multiforme.

Clinical investigation
- The diagnosis is usually based on clinical findings.
- Culture of Coxsackie virus is not straightforward, requiring inoculation of infected material into suckling mice.

Management options
- Supportive care with adequate fluids, anti–inflammatories and rest.
- The condition resolves in seven to ten days and does not recur.

Varicella Zoster
Clinical appearance
- Varicella zoster infection, once established, can be recognised by its classical presentation of unilateral erythema and clusters of vesicles distributed along dermatomes. (Fig 7-5).

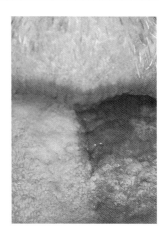

Fig 7-5 Herpes zoster involving the tongue. Note the typical unilateral distribution.

- The vesicles rupture after a few days, become crusted and often coalesce, healing over a period of three weeks, with further vesicles occurring during this time.

Clinical symptoms
- Initial symptoms may be non-specific and can mimic toothache. Patients may also complain of 'electric shock-like' pain.
- As the condition establishes, erythema and clusters of ulcerating vesicles appear. Invariably there is pain, often severe.
- Constitutional upset.

Aetiology
- Reactivation of varicella zoster virus that has remained dormant within dorsal root or cranial nerve ganglia.
- This occurs in older individuals following the waning of immunity to varicella zoster, the infection being contracted during childhood as chicken pox.
- In younger individuals, shingles may be a marker of an immunocompromised host.

Involvement of non-gingival sites
- The classical distribution of the lesions in shingles is that of a belt-like eruption on the trunk.
- In the head and neck region, zoster infections predominantly involve the distribution of the fifth and seventh cranial nerves. The trigeminal nerve is involved in 15% of cases, the ophthalmic division being most frequently affected.

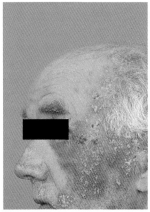

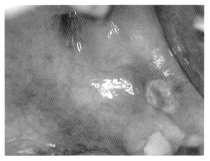

Fig 7-7 Ulceration due to cytomegalovirus infection in a patient with HIV disease.

Fig 7-6 Vesiculation and crusting of facial lesions, distributed across all 3 divisions of the trigeminal nerve.

- Involvement of the maxillary and mandibular divisions of the trigeminal nerve will produce lesions on the facial skin and oral mucosa (Fig 7-6).
- If the ophthalmic division of the trigeminal nerve is involved, corneal ulceration with subsequent scarring may occur.
- Involvement of the geniculate ganglion of the seventh cranial nerve may result in Ramsay Hunt syndrome (lower motor neurone facial palsy, vesicles in the external auditory meatus and sometimes palatal mucosal involvement).

Differential diagnosis
- Herpes simplex infection.
- Myeloproliferative disease.
- Myelosuppressive disease.

Clinical investigation
- The diagnosis is usually made on the basis of clinical features.
- Serological investigation, demonstrating a rise in antibody titre to the virus.
- Cytology.

Management options
- Early treatment with high dose aciclovir, valaciclovir or famciclovir.
- An ophthalmic opinion should be sought if the eye is involved.

- Post herpetic neuralgia may complicate the condition and requires appropriate pain management.

Cytomegalovirus

Localised ulceration due to generalised cytomegalovirus (CMV) infection in HIV/AIDS patients is occasionally seen. Such infection is usually a marker of severe immunosuppression. (Fig 7-7).

CMV associated ulceration of the gingivae appear as non-specific ulceration, with no distinguishing clinical diagnostic features. A history of HIV/AIDS should arouse suspicion, and the diagnosis is confirmed by viral isolation or in situ hybridisation.

Deep Mycoses

The deep mycoses are an uncommon group of infections that rarely involve the oral mucosa or gingivae. These infections may occur particularly in immunocompromised individuals such as HIV/AIDS patients.

Histoplasmosis is usually due to opportunistic infection with Histoplasma capsulatum. This fungal organism is endemic in parts of America, India and Australia. Oral lesions occur usually when the infection is widely disseminated within the host. These lesions not infrequently involve the gingivae and appear as a persistent painful ulcer that may mimic malignant ulceration. Occasionally oral involvement may be the initial presenting sign of the infection.

Diagnosis can be difficult due to the variability of clinical presentation and the lack of specific features. Histological and immunocytochemical investigations are helpful.

Paracoccidiomycosis is a fungal organism found in Brazil and other parts of South America and may produce painful gingival ulceration. The ulceration is often rather granular and mimics pyostomatitis vegetans in appearance.

Other opportunistic deep mycoses that can produce gingival ulceration include Cryptococcus, Coccidiomycosis and Mucormycosis.

A detailed history including ascertaining whether the patient has travelled to those areas where these mycoses are endemic is essential to enable accurate diagnosis of these rare conditions.

Table 7-2 **Clinical features of recurrent aphthous stomatitis**

	Size	Number	Site	Duration	Recurrence Rate
Minor aphthae	5–10mm	<10	Non-keratinised mucosa and dorsum of tongue	7–14 days	Recurrence rates vary. One episode monthly is common.
Major aphthae	>10mm	1–3	No site restriction, but often oropharngeal	Persistent up to 3 months	
Herpetiform aphthae	1–3mm	10–100	No site restriction	10–14 days	

Samaranayake's Essential Microbiology for Dentistry (2002) is a helpful source of reference on the above infective agents.

Recurrent Aphthous Stomatitis
Recurrent aphthous stomatitis is a common condition affecting approximately 20% of the UK population. The condition typically presents in childhood, adolescence and in young adults (Porter, 1998). Ulceration usually occurs on the oral mucosa rather than the gingivae, but gingival involvement occurs in some cases.

Clinical appearance
Aphthous ulcers are round or ovoid in shape, typically have an erythematous periphery and a homogenous white/grey/yellow base.

Three types have been described based on their clinical features (Table 7-2):
• Minor Aphthous Ulceration (80% cases) – (Fig 7-8).
• Major Aphthous Ulceration (15% case) – (Fig 7-9).
• Herpetiform Aphthous Ulceration (5% cases) – (Fig 7-10).

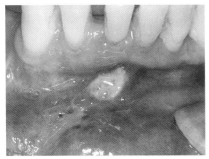

Fig 7-8 Minor aphthous ulceration affecting the alveolar mucosa and gingivae.

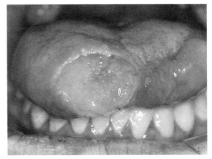

Fig 7-9 Major aphthous ulceration of the tongue.

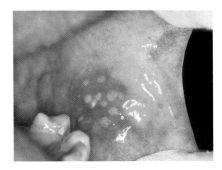

Fig 7-10 Herpetiform ulcers that have started to coalesce.

Clinical symptoms
- Aphthae are painful, major aphthae especially so.
- Herpetiform aphthae may be associated with a mild degree of constitutional upset which can be a source of diagnostic confusion.

Aetiology
Multifactorial and in most patients a cause is not usually identified. The following possibilities should be considered:
- Haematinic deficiency.
- Adult coeliac disease.
- Inflammatory bowel disease (Crohn's disease, ulcerative colitis).
- Lactose intolerance (particularly in Afro-Caribbean patients).
- Other dietary allergies or intolerances.
- Behcet's disease.
- Systemic Lupus erythematosus.
- Reiter's syndrome.
- Bone marrow dysfunction.
- Hormonal – relationship to the pre-luteal phase of menstruation.

Involvement of non-gingival sites
- Aphthous ulcers may occur on any oral mucosal surface.
- Patients with Behcet's disease may also have aphthous type ulceration on their genitalia.

Differential diagnosis
- Traumatic ulceration.
- Underlying systemic disease.
- Behcet's disease.

Clinical investigation
- Full blood count.
- Serum ferritin, folate and B12.
- Biochemical profile, acute phase markers and appropriate immunological investigations, dependent on the clinical features and other laboratory findings (e.g. anti-intrinsic factor and anti-gastric parietal cell antibodies in B12 deficiency).

Management options
- Identification and treatment of underlying/undiagnosed disease.
- Chlorhexidine 0.2% mouthwash.
- Topical anti-inflammatories (Benzydamine hydrochloride).

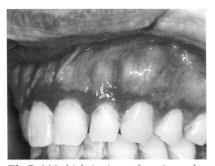 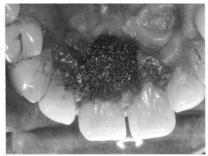

Fig 7-11 Labial gingivae of a patient who developed proliferative veruccous leukoplakia within an area of desquamative gingivitis.

Fig 7-12 Palatal gingival of the patient in Fig 7-11 showing the proliferative veruccous leukoplakia. Squamous cell carcinoma was subsequently identified within the excision specimen.

- Topical corticosteroids (Prednesol or Betnesol mouthrinses).
- Covering agents (Orabase).
- Topical anaesthetic agents (Lidocaine gel).
- In severe cases, systemic corticosteroids ± azathioprine with appropriate monitoring.
- Other agents such as colchicine, thalidomide and immunomodulating drugs may be used in specialist units.

Neoplastic Ulceration

Neoplastic ulceration is an uncommon cause of oral ulceration in general. This is particularly the case with the gingivae. There are various case reports of benign (Tosios, 1993) and metastatic tumours affecting the gingivae, but such occurrences are, however, rare.

Oral malignancy accounts for 1-2% of total human malignancies within the UK. Only 5% of oral malignancies occur on the gingivae. Oral squamous cell carcinoma may arise de novo or from oral premalignant lesions or conditions (Neville, 2002). Rarely malignancy may arise within desquamative gingivitis. (Fig 7-11, 7-12).

Neoplastic pathology presenting as ulceration usually signals malignant rather than benign disease. Most of the malignancies that arise within the gingival tissues are squamous cell carcinomas. Additionally, lymphomas may either present as gingival swelling or ulceration. A brief account of lymphoma can be found in Chapter 8.

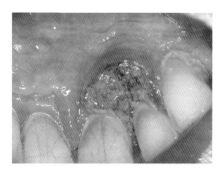

Fig 7-13 Squamous cell carcinoma of the palatal gingiva.

Oral Squamous Cell Carcinoma

Oral squamous cell carcinoma is not commonly found on the gingivae, although it is reported to occur more commonly at this site in Japanese patients. (Laskaris, Scully, 2003).

Clinical appearance
- A persistent, indurated ulcer with a granular base and rolled margin should arouse suspicion. A granular appearance should always be regarded as a sinister clinical finding and demands urgent biopsy. (Fig 7-13).

Clinical symptoms
- Squamous cell carcinoma may be asymptomatic, but if ulcerated will usually cause discomfort. Secondary infection will exacerbate any discomfort.
- Some cases may bleed on minor trauma or even spontaneously.

Aetiology
Whilst the aetiology of oral squamous cell carcinoma is not fully understood, tobacco and alcohol are regarded as the major risk factors.

- Tobacco habits.
- Alcohol.
- Betel nut usage.
- Transformation of premalignant lesions or conditions.
- Poor diet (low in antioxidant content).
- Oncogenic viruses (e.g. Human papilloma virus type 16).
- Ultraviolet radiation (malignant transformation of solar keratoses).

Involvement of non-gingival sites
- Oral squamous cell carcinoma can occur at any site, but in the West most tumours present on the tongue and floor of mouth.

144

- There may be synchronous or metachronous tumours arising elsewhere on the oral mucosa. Approximately 20-30% of patients with oral squamous cell carcinoma will have, or will develop, multiple primary tumours. (Concept of field cancerisation).
- With time there will be local invasion of adjacent tissues as well as development of distant metastases. This will result in additional signs and symptoms including for example, lymphadenopathy, tissue fixity and altered sensation as a result of neural involvement.

Differential diagnosis
- Traumatic ulcer.
- Leukoplakia.
- Erythroplakia.
- Chronic sepsis.
- Lymphoma.
- Histiocytosis X.
- Granulomatous disease.
- Wegener's granulomatosis.
- Pyostomatitis vegetans.

Clinical investigation
- Biopsy is mandatory to establish diagnosis and the exact nature of the tumour, which may influence the definitive therapy.
- Imaging of the primary site, regional lymph nodes (CT, MRI) and chest x-ray.

Management options
Early diagnosis and definitive treatment are most important to maximise the likelihood of a good prognosis.

The major treatment modality is surgical. Radiotherapy may be used either instead of, or additional to, surgical excision, dependent on the clinical scenario.

The therapeutic management of patients with oral squamous cell carcinoma involves a multidisciplinary approach, which includes surgeons, medical oncologists, restorative dentists and appropriate support services.

Metastatic Disease
Metastatic disease of the oral cavity, particularly the gingivae, is uncommon. When it does occur, it usually arises from tumours of the breast (Epstein,

1987), bronchus (Watanabe, 2001) or kidneys. A variety of case reports exist in the literature citing other metastatic tumours presenting on the gingivae, including lymphomas, gastric carcinoma (Shimoyama, 2004), prostatic adenocarcinoma and transitional cell carcinomas of the bladder (Irle, 2001). Usually, gingival involvement of such tumours signals widely disseminated disease.

Further Reading

Alam F, Argiridou AS, Hodgson TA. Primary syphilis remains a cause of oral ulceration. British Dental Journal 2000;189:7,352-354.

Porter SR, Scully CM, Pedersen A. Recurrent aphthous stomatitis. Critical Reviews in Oral Biology and Medicine 1998;9:306-321.

Neville B, Day TA. Oral cancer and precancerous lesions. CA A Cancer Journal for Clinicians 2002;52:195-215.

Laskaris G, Scully C. Periodontal Manifestations of Local and Systemic Diseases. New York: Springer, 2003.

Samaranayake, LP. Essential Microbiology for Dentistry, 2nd edition. Edinburgh: Churchill Livingstone, 2002.

Tosios K, Laskaris G, Eveson J, Scully C. Benign cartilaginous tumour of the gingiva. a case report. International Journal of Oral and Maxillofacial Surgery 1993;22:4,231-233.

Epstein JB, Knowling MA, Le Riche JC. Multiple gingival metastases from angiosarcoma of the breast. Oral Surgery, Oral Medicine, Oral Pathology 1987;64:5,554-557.

Watanabe M, Yasuda K, Tomita K, et al. Lung cancer metastasis to the gingiva. Nihon KokyukiGakkai Zasshi 2001;39:1,50-54.

Shimoyama S, Seto Y, Aoki F, et al. Gastric cancer with metastasis to the gingiva. Journal of Gastroenterology and Hepatology 2004;19:7,831-835.

Irle C. Metastatic transitional cell carcinoma of the urinary bladder presenting as a mandibular gingival swelling. Journal of Periodontology 2001;72:5,688-690.

Chapter 8

Generalised Gingival Ulceration

Aim

The aim of this chapter is to detail those clinical entities that may present as widespread or multiple areas of gingival ulceration.

Outcome

Having read this chapter, the reader should be able to formulate a differential diagnosis in cases of generalised gingival ulceration. They should be aware of the extra-oral manifestations of associated conditions and request and interpret those investigations that will assist definitive diagnosis so facilitating effective clinical management. Table 8-1 summarises the conditions discussed in this chapter.

Vesicles and Bullae

A chapter specifically devoted to vesicular lesions cannot be justified, and therefore some pointers towards their investigation are provided briefly here. The most likely causes of gingival or mucosal vesicles are:

1. Viral infection
2. Trauma, which may be thermal, chemical or mechanical
3. Vesicullo-bullous disease such as mucous membrane (cicatricial) pemphigoid.

In the case of viral lesions, explore the history for a prodrome and check for lymphadenopathy (Fig 1-6) and pyrexia. If trauma is a cause this should be evident from the history, and fluid collected from the vesicle will be inflammatory in nature, with an absence of systemic signs of infection. Vesiculobullous diseases are dealt with in detail in Chapters 7 and 8.

Mucocutaneous Disease

Pemphigoid

Pemphigoid is an autoimmune vesiculobullous disease that manifests with subepithelial bulla formation as a result of the production of antibodies

Table 8-1 **Summary - generalised gingival ulceration**

Major Categories	Sub Categories	Frequency of Condition	Management Setting
Mucocutaneous disease	Mucous membrane pemphigoid	Uncommon/rare	Referral to specialist units for treatment, monitoring and management of possible extra-oral manifestations.
	Pemphigus	Rare	Referral to specialist units – this is a serious condition that may be life-threatening in some cases.
	Lichen planus	A common condition but very rarely produces generalised gingival ulceration.	Severe recalcitrant cases should be referred for specialist assessment.
Haematological	Leukaemias	Uncommon	The condition itself is clearly managed by haematologists. Oral hygiene measures can be undertaken in primary care. Management of the oral mucosal manifestations of chemotherapy/ radio-therapy should be managed in specialist units.

Major Categories	Sub Categories	Frequency of Condition	Management Setting
Lymphomas	Uncommon	As for the leukaemias	
Other haematological disease (e.g. myelosuppressive states)	Rare	As for the leukaemias	
Infections	Primary herpetic gingivostomatitis – See Chapter 4	Uncommon More usually associated with erythema than generalised gingival ulceration.	Supportive measures and antiviral agents such as aciclovir which are only of real value if therapy is instituted at onset or very early in the course of the disease

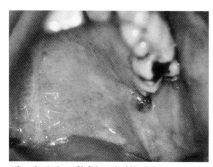

Fig 8-1 Small blood-filled blister that could be mistaken for a traumatic blister.

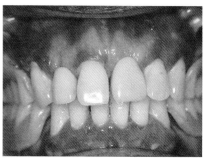

Fig 8-2 Mucous membrane pemphigoid presenting as desquamative gingivitis.

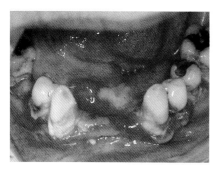

Fig 8-3 Desquamative gingivitis with erosions.

directed to the basement membrane zone of the epithelium. The disease is usually seen in patients over 50 years of age and is twice as common in females (Chan, 2002). There are two major variants of the condition:

- Mucous Membrane Pemphigoid - predominantly mucosal involvement.
- Bullous pemphigoid - predominantly cutaneous involvement.

Clinical appearance
- The manifestations of mucous membrane pemphigoid often commence in the mouth and on occasions may be confined to the oral mucosa. (Fig 8-1).
- Although oral lesions rarely precede skin lesions in bullous pemphigoid, oral mucosal disease may be a feature of this variant.
- The main periodontal manifestation of mucous membrane pemphigoid is desquamative gingivitis (Fig 8-2), which may be the only oral feature of the condition (see Chapter 4). Shallow erosions may occur in desquamative gingivitis associated with vesiculobullous disease (Fig 8-3) (Richards, 2005).

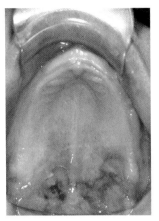

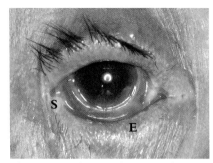

Fig 8-5 Ocular involvement showing entropion (E) and symblepharon (S).

Fig 8-4 Typical palatal erosions in mucous membrane pemphigoid.

- Serum anti-basement membrane antibodies can be identified in 80% of cases of bullous and 60% of cases of mucous membrane pemphigoid.
- Desquamative gingivitis may also occur in pemphigus/lichen planus/DLE.
- Extra-oral manifestations of mucous membrane pemphigoid are problematical due to scarring and subsequent scar contraction. Common sites of involvement include the eyes, genitals and oesophagus.
- Rarely there may be an association with internal malignancy.

Clinical symptoms
- Soreness is the principal symptom often accompanied by bleeding on brushing.
- The discomfort may be such that the patient cannot tolerate flavouring oils used in many dentifrices.
- Patients may also be concerned at the appearance of the gingivae, which may be fiery red.
- Patients may complain of intra-oral blistering, but the blisters often go unnoticed. It is only when they burst to produce painful ulceration that the problem is drawn to the patient's attention. The blisters may persist for several days, but often rupture within a few hours.
- Blistering and subsequent ulceration may be provoked by the ingestion of abrasive foods.

Aetiology
- Pemphigoid is an autoimmune disease associated with the production of antibodies to the basement membrane zone of the epithelium.

Involvement of non-gingival sites
- Mucous membrane pemphigoid, as the name suggests, can affect any mucosal surface. Intra-orally the distal hard palate and soft palate are commonly affected as the bolus of food is pushed up into this location prior to deglutition. Clinically the appearance is one of shallow irregular ulceration, with an erythematous and sometimes haemorrhagic border (Fig 8-4). There may be keratosis peripheral to the ulceration representing scar tissue that frequently accompanies healing.
- Extra-oral involvement may involve the oesophagus, which can become stenosed producing dysphagia.
- Genital lesions – these may be very disabling.
- Ocular lesions - these are often initially insidious and may affect up to 60% of patients. They are potentially serious, compromising sight. The eyelids may become sore as a result of blistering and subsequent ulceration. Subsequently the eyelids turn inwards due to scar contraction (entropion). Conjunctival scarring also occurs producing a symblepharon (scarring and fusion of the tarsal and bulbar conjunctiva) (Fig 8-5).
- Nasal lesions may occur, manifesting as bleeding and crusting of the nasal mucosa.
- Cutaneous involvement may occur in mucous membrane pemphigoid.

Differential diagnosis
Clinically, desquamative gingivitis that is ulcerated is suggestive of a vesiculobullous aetiology rather than lichen planus, which is the most common cause of desquamative gingivitis. The distribution of the lesions both within the oral cavity and extra-orally is helpful in arriving at a diagnosis. Differential diagnoses include:
- Pemphigus.
- Linear IgA disease.
- Erythema multiforme.
- Traumatic blistering.
- Epidermolysis bullosa acquisita
- Dermatitis herpetiformis.

Clinical investigation
- The gold standard for diagnosis is direct immunofluorescence of an unfixed mucosal biopsy, which should be taken from a new or nearly new

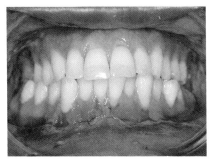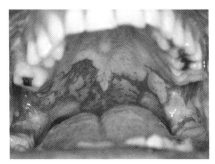

Fig 8-6 Pemphigus vulgaris involving the gingivae, producing a desquamative gingivitis with areas of erosion and haemorrhage.

Fig 8-7 Pemphigus vulgaris involving the palate

lesion. It is most important to include a margin of perilesional tissue. Linear deposits of IgG and C3 are characteristically identified at the basement membrane level in mucous membrane pemphigoid.
- Routine histopathological examination should also be undertaken.
- Circulating anti-basement membrane zone antibodies can be identified by indirect immunofluorescence, but this is a much less sensitive test, being positive in approximately 60% of patients, dependent on the method employed.
- Clinically a positive Nikolsky sign may be elicited (bulla formation or propagation on trauma).

Management options
- An ophthalmic opinion in all cases of mucous membrane pemphigoid is mandatory – untreated eye disease has potentially serious consequences.
- Topical corticosteroids if disease is limited to the mouth.
- More severe or widespread disease may necessitate the use of systemic corticosteroid therapy possibly associated with a steroid–sparing drug such as azathioprine. Dapsone, mycophenolate mofetil or tacrolimus may also have a therapeutic role. Such drugs should only be used in specialist units.
- Referral to other specialties as demanded by the sites of involvement.

Pemphigus
Pemphigus is an intraepithelial autoimmune bullous disorder that is less common but potentially more serious than pemphigoid. It presents in various forms:
- P. vulgaris - usually the variant that involves the oral mucosa and is detailed below.

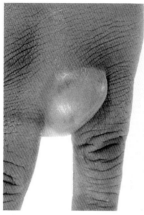

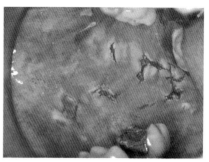

Fig 8-9 Slit-like ulcers in oral mucosal pemphigus.

Fig 8-8 Flaccid bulla in cutaneous pemphigus.

- P. vegetans.
- P. erythematosus.
- P. foliaceous – this variant does not affect the oral mucosa.

Clinical appearance
- Mucosal involvement is common and often precedes cutaneous involvement. Oral mucosal involvement may be the initial presenting sign, particularly desquamative gingivitis, perhaps several months ahead of other sites (Fig 8-6, 8-7).
- Blisters are often flaccid rather than the tense blisters seen in pemphigoid and are fragile as they are thin-walled (intra-epithelial) (Fig 8-8).
- On rupturing, the blisters may leave large shallow erosions with ragged edges, or discrete slit-like ulcers with jagged margins, often surrounded by white mucosa (Fig 8-9).
- Blisters occur at sites of trauma – palatal involvement therefore is frequent.
- Desquamative gingivitis is common and may be the only presenting sign. It may be associated with gingival erosions as in pemphigoid.

Clinical symptoms
- Patients will complain of ulceration and associated pain, inflamed gingivae and on occasions blistering at mucosal and cutaneous sites. In the early stages, however, patients may be unaware of blister formation.
- The symptoms are very similar to those described for pemphigoid.

Aetiology
- An autoimmune disease associated with the production of antibodies to intercellular cement of mucosal and skin surfaces. In pemphigus vulgaris these are usually antibodies to desmoglein 3, a transmembrane desmosomal glycoprotein.

Involvement of non-gingival sites
- Many cases presenting on the oral mucosa remain localised to the mouth, however with time some cases involve the skin and other mucosal sites such as the genitalia.
- Some patients will develop extra-oral lesions rapidly following the appearance of the oral lesions. It is important to inform patients that they must seek immediate advice should extra-oral involvement develop. Patients are at risk from fluid and electrolyte disturbances due to the loss of fluid from the ruptured blisters, together with consequent infection.

Differential diagnosis
- Pemphigoid – the skin lesions in bullous pemphigoid tend to involve the upper limbs whereas those of pemphigus occur more usually on the trunk.
- The differential diagnosis is otherwise as that detailed for pemphigoid.

Clinical investigation
- A positive Nikolsky sign as a result of widespread acantholysis (detachment of keratinocytes) can be demonstrated clinically by gentle trauma to an area of clinically uninvolved mucosa or skin, which results in bulla formation.
- IgG and C3 are demonstrable intercellularly by direct immunofluorescence.
- Serum anti-intercellular cement antibody levels correlate with disease activity and can be identified by indirect immunofluorescence.
- If there is clinical suspicion of occult malignant disease (usually lymphoma, leukaemia, thymoma or gastrointestinal malignancy) appropriate investigations should be undertaken. (paraneoplastic pemphigus, Sklavounou, Laskaris, 1998).

Management options
- If the lesions are confined to the oral mucosa, then local management with topical steroids is the preferred choice.
- If the lesions are unresponsive to local measures or there is extra-oral involvement, then systemic corticosteroid therapy is indicated. This may be combined with azathioprine as a steroid sparing agent, and is likely to have to be given long term.

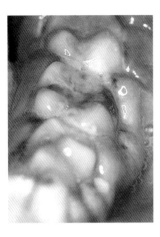

Fig 8-10 Hyperplastic gingivae in acute myeloid leukaemia.

- Multidisciplinary management is the norm.
- Pemphigus can be a fatal condition. Prompt and effective management is of paramount importance.

Lichen Planus
Although lichen planus frequently manifests as erosions on the oral mucosa, erosive lesions on the gingivae are uncommon and ulceration at this site is more suggestive of vesiculobullous pathology. A full account of lichen planus can be found in Chapter 4.

Haematological Disease

The Leukaemias
The leukaemias represent a range of serious haematological disorders that arise as a result of abnormal maturation or proliferation of the various white blood cell lines. There are both acute and chronic forms and any of the white cell types may be involved, but most frequently it is the lymphoid or myeloid lines.

The acute leukaemias are more likely to have oral manifestations than the chronic variants, and on occasions, it is these manifestations that may be the first presenting sign of the disease.

Clinical features
- Gingival hyperplasia and swelling due to leukaemic cell infiltration (Fig 8-10). This may be seen in 20-30% of patients with acute myeloid

leukaemia, although rather less frequently in cases of acute lymphoblastic leukaemia (2%), a condition that is most prevalent in childhood.
- The gingivae appear erythematous and may bleed easily on mild trauma or spontaneously as a result of thrombocytopaenia.
- Specific infections such as necrotising ulcerative gingivitis (NUG), herpes simplex or candidosis may occur.
- Rarely there may be rapid loss of periodontal support as a consequence of malignant cell infiltration of the periodontal ligament.
- Chronic leukaemias are much less likely to present with periodontal manifestations.

Aetiology
- Malignant clonal proliferation of white blood cells.
- A variety of cytogenetic abnormalities are identifiable in the leukaemic cells (e.g. the Philadelphia chromosome).
- The malignant cells displace the non-malignant cell progenitors, resulting in anaemias and platelet depletion.
- Infection may result as a consequence of non-functional or depleted immunocompetent cells.

Involvement of non-gingival sites
- The patient is often acutely ill and may have features of severe anaemia including breathlessness.
- Oral mucosal purpura.
- Oral ulceration.
- Mucosal pallor due to anaemia.
- Candidosis.
- Lymphadenopathy.
- Cutaneous involvement.
- Bruising.
- Hepatosplenomegaly.

Differential diagnosis
- Other myeloproliferative or myelosuppressive disease.
- Immunodeficiency states.
- Histiocytosis X.
- Plasma cell gingivitis.
- Inflammatory gingival enlargements.
- Pyostomatitis vegetans.

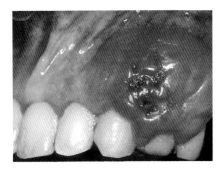

Fig 8-11 Non-Hodgkins lymphoma.

Clinical investigation
- Incisional biopsy of involved tissue.
- Appropriate haematological investigations including full and differential white count, blood film and bone marrow aspirate and biopsy.
- Immunophenotyping.

Management options
- The leukaemia will be managed by the haematologist, usually with combination chemotherapy.
- Local measures include scrupulous oral hygiene and adjunctive topical antiseptic agents.
- Painful oral ulceration may be managed by topical anti-inflammatories, anaesthetics and covering agents.
- Management of the local side-effects of chemotherapy and radiotherapy.

The Lymphomas
Most lymphomas are B cell tumours and rarely affect the gingivae. Hodgkins lymphomas are less prevalent in the orofacial region than non-Hodgkins lymphomas, the latter presenting in the oropharyngeal region in approximately 10% of cases. The lymphomas seen in the oral cavity may either represent metastatic deposits or primary tumours that may be maltomas (mucosa-associated lymphoid tissue lymphomas). The classification of lymphomas is complex and beyond the scope of this book.

Clinical features
- Non-Hodgkins lymphomas may present as a painless swelling on the gingivae, usually soft in texture (Fig 8-11). The clinical appearance often does not arouse suspicion of sinister pathology, particularly in the early stages.
- They may mimic dental or periodontal sepsis.

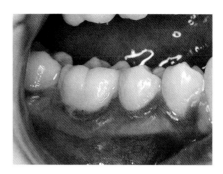

Fig 8-12 Gingival ulceration adjacent to the lower right first molar tooth in a neutropaenic patient.

- The mucosal surface of the lymphoma deposit varies in colour from clinically normal to erythematous and it may occasionally ulcerate and become painful.
- Tooth mobility may occur.

Aetiology
- Unclear, but some are associated with viral infections.
- An increased frequency of lymphoma occurs in association with certain autoimmune conditions including Sjogren's syndrome (MALTomas).
- Certain immunodeficiency syndromes predispose to lymphomas (ataxia telangiectasia; Wiskott Aldrich syndrome).
- Non-malignant disease involving the lymphoreticular system also appears to be associated with the development of lymphomas in the long term.

Involvement of non-gingival sites
- Waldeyer's ring may be involved intra-orally, particularly when there is gastrointestinal tract involvement.
- Rarely, oral mucosal ulceration may occur.
- Lymphadenopathy.

Differential diagnosis
- Dental or periodontal sepsis.
- Inflammatory swellings.
- Fibroepithelial hyperplasia.
- Non lymphoreticular tumours.
- Other metastatic deposits.

Clinical investigation
- Biopsy is mandatory.

- Immunocytochemical studies will be required to identify the appropriate cell markers that facilitate classification of the lymphoma.

Management options
- Referral to haematology for further investigation and staging.
- Chemotherapy and radiotherapy.

Other Haematological Conditions

Various other diseases occurring as a result of abnormal bone marrow function, can also produce ulcerative conditions that affect the gingivae and the oral mucosa. These include, agranulocytosis, neutropaenic states (Fig. 8-12) and myelodysplasia. (Chapple et al 1999).

Further Reading

Chan LS, Ahmad AR, Anhalt GJ et al. The first international consensus on mucous membrane pemphigoid: Definition, diagnostic criteria, pathogenic factors, medical treatment and prognostic indicators. Archives of Dermatology 2002;138:3,370-379.

Richards A. Desquamative gingivitis and its management. Perio in Practice Today 2005;3: 183-190.

Sklavounou A, Laskaris G. Paraneoplastic pemphigus: a review. Oral Oncology 1998; 34:6,437-440.

Chapple ILC, Saxby MS, Murray J. Gingival haemorrhage, myelodysplastic syndromes and acute myeloid leukaemia. Journal of Periodontology 1999:70,1247-1253.

Chapter 9
Localised Gingival Recession

Aim

This chapter aims to outline the principal causes of localised gingival recession, including those associated with underlying systemic disease.

Outcome

At the end of this chapter the reader will be aware of the limited range of conditions that give rise to localised gingival recession and be able to recognise when referral may be prudent. Table 9-1 lists the causes of localised gingival recession. Some of these conditions are common and are best managed in the primary care sector, whilst others are less common and patients should be referred for further investigation and specialist therapy.

Classification of Localised Recession Defects

There have been several proposed classification systems to enable clinical documentation of local recession defects. Whilst not the most appropriate for diagnostic purposes, the most frequently used system is currently that proposed by Miller (Fig 9-1). This system was designed primarily to indicate the likelihood of successful management using periodontal plastic surgery procedures to correct recession defects. A practical and novel diagnostic recording system based upon clinical measurements is proposed below:
1. Measurement of the length of the recession in mm from the CEJ to the base of the defect (L1, L2 for 1mm, 2mm etc – Fig 9-2a)
2. Measurement of the width of the defect in mm at its widest aspect mesio-distally (W1, W2 for 1mm, 2mm etc – Fig 9-2b)
3. Specification of the number of teeth involved (T1, T2 etc – Fig 9-2c)
4. Identification of whether the extent of the defect is superior (S) or inferior (I) to the mucogingival junction (MGJ – Fig 9-2d).

Therefore, in Fig 9-3 the defect at LR1 would be annotated as L5/W2/T1/I and at LL1 as L3/W2/T1/S.

Table 9-1 **Localised gingival recession**

Condition	Sub Category Nature	Incidence	Manage/ Refer
Developmental defects	Dehiscence	common	manage/refer
	Fenestration	common	manage/refer
	Anatomical tooth position	common	manage/refer
Traumatic defects	Class II division 2 incisor relationship and gingival stripping	common	refer
	Conscious self-induced mutilation (gingivitis artefacta)	rare	refer
	Subconscious self-induced mutilation	rare	manage
Inflammatory defects	Localised aggressive periodontitis	common	manage/refer
	Peridontal-endodontic lesions	common	manage
	Localised chronic periodontitis	common	manage
Defects associated with underlying systematic disease	Linear Morphoea	uncommon	refer
	Histiocytosis X	uncommon	refer
	Necrotising periodontitis (HIV)	uncommon	refer
	Necrotising stomatitis (HIV)	uncommon	refer
Drug-induced lesions	Cocaine	uncommon	refer
	Aspirin	uncommon	manage

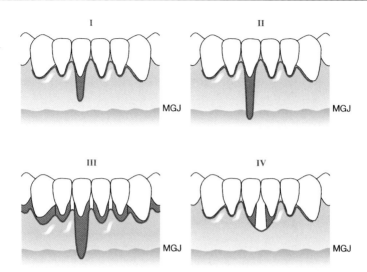

Fig 9-1 Miller's classification of recession defects. I – Marginal tissue recession not extending to MGJ. No loss of interdental bone or soft tissue. II – Marginal tissue recession extends to or beyond MGJ. No loss of interdental bone or soft tissue. III – Marginal tissue recession extends to or beyond MGJ. Loss of interdental bone or soft tissue is apical to the CEJ, but coronal to the apical extent of the marginal tissue recession. IV – As for III but loss of interdental bone or soft tissue is apical to the CEJ and extends to a level beyond the apical-most extent of marginal tissue recession.

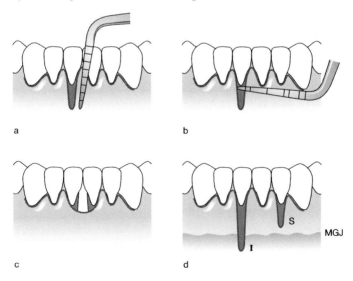

Fig 9-2 Proposed diagnostic coding/notation system for recording recession defects.

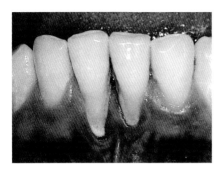

Fig 9-3 Recession defect (Stillman's cleft) affecting LR1 (L4/W2/T1/I) and LL1 (L3/W2/T1/S). Had the interdental papilla been missing between LR1 and LL1, the defect class would have been L4/W6/T2/I .

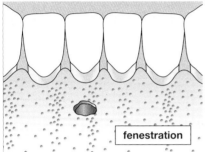
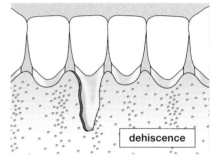

Fig 9-4 Schematic diagram illustrating a bony fenestration and dehiscence affecting LR1.

Developmental Conditions

Dehiscence and Fenestration

Two classical developmental anomalies can predispose to localised recession defects sometimes referred to as 'Stillman's clefts' (Fig 9-3). These are illustrated in Fig 9-4:

- Dehiscence – the absence of a 'window' of bone at the facial or oral surface of a tooth (normally buccal/labial plate), i.e. the alveolar margin remains intact.
- Fenestration – a 'V'-shaped defect involving the alveolar margin and extending apically.

A significant amount of the blood supply to the gingivae arrives via the periosteum and an absence of periosteal blood supply renders the gingival marginal tissue less able to resist trauma and recurrent inflammation (plaque-induced), without loss of marginal epithelium and subsequent recession. The teeth most commonly affected are lower incisors and upper canines. Contrary to popular belief, there is no evidence for a direct effect from 'fraenal pull' as

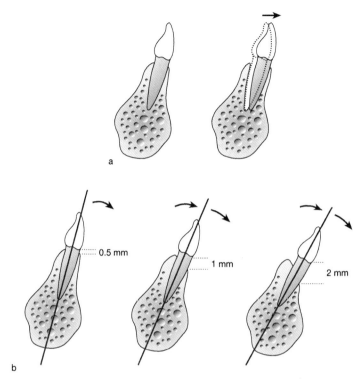

Fig 9-5 a) Incisors positioned labially within the alveolus relative to the ideal, thereby leaving a thin labial bone plate. b) Incisors proclined in a compensatory manner in a patient with a mild class II skeletal base, thereby reducing the overbite and compromising the integrity of the labial crestal bone.

the fraenum rarely carries muscle fibres (Watts 2000). However, the fraenum may interfere with plaque control around lower incisors where the labial bone plate is thin, or there is an underlying anatomical bone defect. Prominent fraena may therefore contribute to the development of recession following repeated episodes of gingival inflammation, secondary to an inability to maintain plaque control in the area.

Anatomical Tooth Position
On occasions the lower incisors develop in a position that is more labial than 'ideal' and/or are also proclined, further reducing the thickness of labial crestal bone, or indeed its coronal extent (Fig 9-5). The overlying gingivae appear extremely thin and delicate (Fig 9-6) and are prone to recession if marginal plaque control is less than ideal.

Box 9-1 **The Akerly classification of traumatic incisal relationships. Taken from Heasman, Preshaw and Robertson, 2004.**

Class 1	Lower incisors impinge on the palatal mucosa, posterior to the palatal gingival margins of the maxillary anterior teeth.
Class II	Lower incisors occlude onto the palatal gingival margins of the maxillary anterior teeth.
Class III	A deep traumatic overbite (Class II div 2 incisor relationship) with shearing of the mandibular labial gingivae.
Class IV	Lower incisors occlude with the palatal surfaces of the upper incisors, leading to tooth wear by attrition.

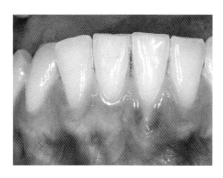

Fig 9-6 Delicate tissue biotype prone to recession due to plaque-induced inflammation and toothbrush trauma.

Traumatic Defects
Class II division 1 or 2 incisor relationship with gingival stripping.

Clinical appearance
Gingival stripping may arise in a Class II division 1 or 2 incisor relationship. Akerly classified such incisor relationships from an orthodontic perspective (Box 9-1) but in periodontal terms, Akerly Class II and III relationships are the most significant and very difficult to manage (see Heasman, Preshaw and Robertson 2004). Localised recession defects affecting one or all of the incisor teeth may be evident:
- palatally to the upper incisors and caused by a traumatic overbite of the lower incisor edges against the palatal gingival margins (Fig 9-7). This may arise in a class II division 1 incisor relationship, where the overjet is

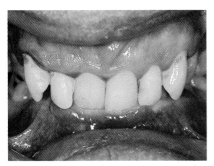

Fig 9-7 A Class II division 2 incisor relationship with trauma to the lower labial gingivae (see blanching of lower gingival margins) (Akerly Class III).

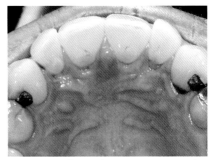

Fig 9-8 A Class II division 2 incisor relationship with trauma to the palatal gingivae of the maxillary incisors (Akerley Class II).

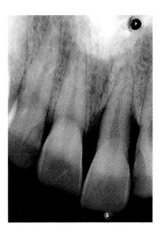

Fig 9-9 Radiograph demonstrating over-eruption of UL 1 post-periodontal bone loss and a crescentic pattern of bone loss indicative of occlusal trauma.

increased and the overbite is complete, or in a class II division 2 incisor relationship with a complete overbite.

• labially to the lower incisors and caused by the incisal edges of the upper anterior teeth occluding against the labial gingival margin (Fig 9-8). This arises in a class II division 2-incisor relationship.

Clinical symptoms
• Pain on eating/incising.
• Soreness/ulceration of the gingival margin.
• Recession.
• Aesthetic concerns related to the anterior tooth position or more generally the malocclusion (especially if there is a large skeletal component).

167

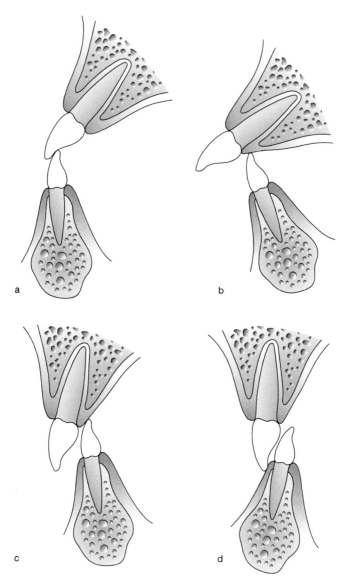

Fig 9-10 Schematic representation of a) a 'stable' incisor relationship, with the incisal edge of the lower teeth against the palatal cingulum rest of the upper incisors; b) an unstable Class II div 1 relationship with trauma to the palatal gingival margins; c) an unstable Class II div 2 relationship with trauma to the palatal gingival margins; d) an unstable Class II div 2 relationship with trauma to the labial mandibular gingival margins.

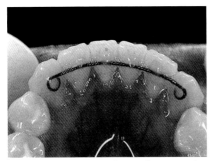

Fig 9-11 A twist wire and composite splint to permanently retain the lower incisors post-orthodontic therapy.

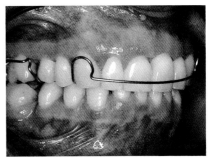

Fig 9-12 An upper removable retainer designed for night time use to maintain a stable incisor relationship.

Aetiology
- Unstable incisor relationship due to skeletal relationship of mandible to maxilla or habitual (thumb sucking), resulting in retroclination of lower incisors and proclination of uppers.
- Unstable incisor relationship due to loss of periodontal support (periodontal disease) and incisor tooth movement or over-eruption (Fig 9-9).

Involvement of non-gingival sites
None.

Differential diagnosis
None. The key diagnostic decision is whether there is historical or currently active periodontitis.

Clinical investigation
- Study models to examine the incisor relationship (Fig 9-10).
- Radiographs.
- Orthodontic opinion.
- Incisor set up on models for orthodontic realignment, as a diagnostic procedure.
- Incisor set up (Kesling set up) for a restorative solution (e.g. 'Dahl' appliance – see Noble, Kellet and Chapple 2004).

Management options
- Establishing a stable incisor relationship by orthodontic means is the ideal solution, but frequently requires lengthy therapy and permanent retention, either fixed (Fig-9-11) or removable (Fig 9-12).

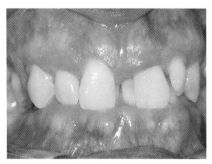

Fig 9-13a Class II incisor relationship with traumatic overbite causing palatal gingival stripping.

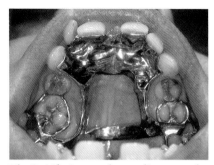

Fig 9-13b An overlay appliance can be made and fitted prior to reduction of the lower incisor edges, which are reduced when the appliance is fitted, the chrome thereby occupying the resultant space.

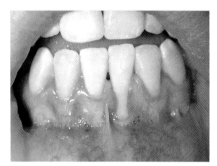

Fig 9-14a Localised recession defect, which was likely to worsen with orthodontic realignment of the lower incisors, which involved their proclination. Oral hygiene was excellent prior to surgery.

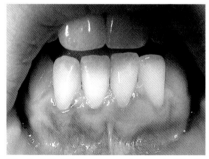

Fig 9-14b The same patient as in Fig 9-14a, post-connective tissue graft surgery and orthodontic treatment.

- A 'Dahl' appliance may be of value to intrude/retrocline the lower incisors and encourage over-eruption of posterior teeth, thereby separating the upper incisors from the lower labial gingivae.
- An overlay appliance to prevent further trauma (Fig 9-13).
- If the recession defect is localised, pre-orthodontic treatment by connective tissue grafting can improve aesthetics and hygiene prior to establishing a stable anterior tooth relationship (Fig 9-14).

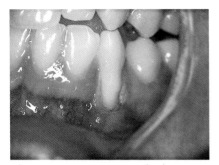

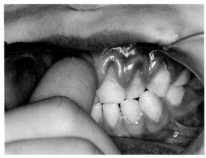

Fig 9-15 Factitious injury also known as gingivitis artefacta, caused by fingernail picking of the gingival margin LL3. Note the marginal keratosis and absence of plaque, consistent with repeated trauma. The patient had previously exfoliated her LR3.

Fig 9-16 Gingivitis artefacta in a child demonstrating how the trauma was caused.

Conscious Self-Mutilation (see also Chapter 7)

Clinical appearance

- Localised recession defects, which appear plaque free.
- Marginal keratosis indicates chronic trauma (Fig 9-15).
- Notched recession defects (Fig 9-16).
- Absence of traumatic incisor relationship.

Clinical symptoms

- Remarkably, pain is not usually a complaint.
- Itching gums may indicate psychiatric morbidity.
- Aesthetic concerns completely out of proportion to the true size/nature of the problem may indicate an obsessive-compulsive disorder.
- Patient is often symptom-free and brought by a concerned relative/parent or referred by their dental surgeon.

Aetiology

- Habitual (Fig 9-16). This may arise in patients with a learning disability, or as in the illustrated case, in children where the maxilla is the main focus.
- Attention-seeking/psychiatric morbitidy (Fig 9-17). Severe forms are known as Munchausen's syndrome, where patients deliberately self-mutilate to seek medical or surgical intervention. The patient in Fig 9-17 suffered from an obsessive-compulsive disorder and traumatised his gingival margin UR1 with scissors.

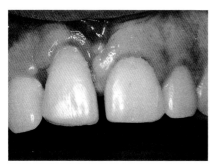

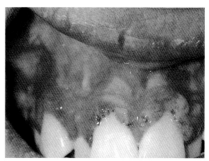

Fig 9-17 A 17-year-old male clinically diagnosed with obsessive-compulsive disorder.

Fig 9-18 A 14-year-old girl with extensive annular and exophytic gingival lesions atypical of 'artefacta'. (The patient submitted to several blood investigations and repeat biopsies before a factitious cause was suspected. Munchausen's syndrome remained a likely diagnosis for this patient at the time of this book going to press).

Involvement of non-gingival sites
- Habitual self-mutilation in its mildest form can frequently involve the buccal mucosa or lips (from habitual tissue chewing or biting), or indeed any other part of the body.
- Attention-seeking may involve ulcerative lesions like those illustrated in Fig 9-18, but arising anywhere on the oral mucosa; the tongue is a common site. Psychiatric morbidity may again result in trauma to any part of the body. The 17-year-old male illustrated in Fig 9-17 also mutilated the enamel of his UR1 using a metal file.

Differential diagnosis
- Toothbrush trauma.
- Stillman's cleft.
- Localised periodontitis ± occlusal trauma.

Clinical investigation
- An important test in arriving at a differential diagnosis is to disclose the teeth to eliminate a plaque-induced cause. In self-mutilation, the constant agitation removes plaque and generally the tooth surface is plaque free.

Management options
- Habitual self-mutilation – frequently drawing the habit to the patient's

172

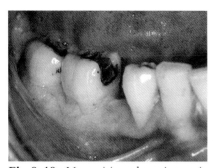

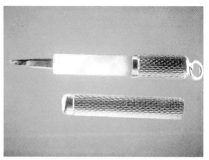

Fig 9-19a Necrotising ulcerative peri-odontitis caused by trauma from a silver tooth pick. The interproximal and marginal epithelium was denuded, along with the local periosteum, which led subsequently to bone sequestration.

Fig 9-19b The silver tooth pick used to inadvertently create the recession/ulcerative defect LR 67.

attention may be sufficient to break the habit or the fabrication of a soft occlusal guard for night use may help.

- Discussion with the patient and/or parents. The female in Fig 9-18 had very low self-esteem. She underwent two biopsies over a period of two years and several blood investigations to eliminate gastrointestinal pathology (e.g. Coeliac disease) before a diagnosis by exclusion was made. Discussion in the absence of her parents brought the true diagnosis to light (the patient then chose to tell her parents). Munchausen's syndrome was a differential diagnosis in this case.

- Attention-seeking – letting the patient know that you are aware of the cause and a frank and open discussion with them about their habit may be sufficient to stop the habit. It may be necessary to have a discussion without any parent or guardian present (but witnessed by a member of your staff), in case the parent/guardian is contributory to the problem and for reasons of confidentiality. Professional counselling may be needed, or medical/psychiatric intervention where Munchausen's syndrome is suspected.

- Psychiatric disease requires psychiatric referral, usually through the patient's medical practitioner.

Subconscious Self-Mutilation

Factitious injury can arise from a habitual practice, of which the patient is unaware. It generally arises in situations where a patient is obsessed with cleaning a particular interproximal site and the patient unwittingly and

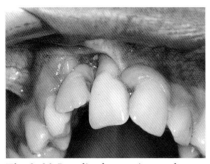

Fig 9-20 Localised recession and scarring affecting UR12, due to linear morphoea/localised scleroderma in a 14-year-old-female.

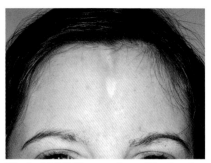

Fig 9-21 Midline scaring of forehead, a 'coupe de sabre' in the same patient as illustrated in Fig 9-20, which was hidden by a fringe.

unintentionally causes local trauma. The most common example would be a localised acute inflammatory swelling caused by inappropriate use of dental floss or tape. However, more significant ulcerative/recession lesions can also arise. The patient illustrated in Fig 9-19 created a necrotising ulcerative lesion LR67 using a silver-plated toothpick to perform interproximal plaque control. The marginal alveolar bone sequestrated and subsequent healing by secondary intention was very slow.

Inflammatory/Infective Conditions
The following lesions are beyond the scope of this text and are discussed in more detail in other books within this Periodontology series.
- Inflammatory defects.
- Localised aggressive periodontitis (see Clerehugh, Tugnait and Chapple, 2004, and Heasman, Preshaw and Robertson, 2004).
- Periodontal-endodontic lesions (see Noble, Kellett and Chapple 2004).
- Localised chronic periodontitis (see Heasman, Preshaw and Robertson 2004).

Defects Associated with Underlying Systemic Disease

Linear Morphoea (Localised Scleroderma)
Clinical appearance
- Localised midline gingival retraction (Fig 9-20).
- Gingival scarring (white appearance to gingivae).

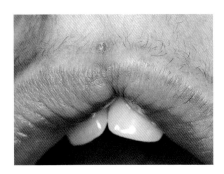

Fig 9-22 Midline lip notching/retraction in the patient from Fig 9-20.

Clinical symptoms
- Receding gums.
- Root sensitivity.
- Aesthetic concerns.
- Concerns over tooth loss.

Aetiology
Localised scleroderma is a rare condition also referred to as 'Morphoea' and is predominantly a cutaneous disease. It is believed to have a genetic basis or, alternately, to arise following trauma. The case illustrated in Figs 9-20 to 9-22 was a 14-year-old girl referred for connective tissue grafting to the UR12 area, following the development of localised recession. Careful examination revealed a midline forehead scar hidden beneath the girl's fringe. Given the midline position and cutaneous nature of the scarring, surgery was ruled out as the chance of a graft or rotational flap re-vascularising was minimal and aggressive treatment deemed more likely to make the situation worse. Laser surgery to the lip prior to the diagnosis did indeed make the lip retraction more severe (Baxter et al, 2001).

Involvement of non-gingival sites
- 'Coupe de sabre' (linear cut of the sword) – scarring which may affect the forehead (Fig 9-21).
- Midline lip notching/lip retraction (Fig 9-22).
- Scarring elsewhere, but limited to the skin.

Differential diagnosis
- Bony dehiscence.
- Tissue loss following trauma.
- Localised periodontitis.
- Self-mutilation (gingivitis artefacta).

Clinical investigation
- Careful history to eliminate trauma.
- Family history.
- Medical history.
- Scarring elsewhere on body.
- Clinical examination to eliminate true pocketing/periodontitis.
- Extra-oral examination for evidence of related scarring.

Management options
The periodontal condition can be managed conservatively with non-surgical methods. In the case described, it was so-managed for four years, but when the patient reached 16 years of age and aesthetics became an important factor in her life, she opted for extraction and prosthetic replacement of UR12. A lip split and contour revision using autogenous fat injections was also performed and future fixed prostheses are planned (+ implant retainers).

Histiocytosis-X

Three forms of histiocytosis-X are described:
1. Unifocal eosinophilic granuloma (solitary).
2. Multifocal eosinophilic granuloma (Hand-Schuller-Christian disease).
3. Progressive/disseminated histiocytosis (Letterer-Siwe disease).

Eosinophilic Granuloma
Clinical appearance
Mandible more commonly than maxilla and often posterior sites. There may be buccal swelling, which may appear exophytic, deep pocketing and gingival bleeding or it may present as a localised gingival recession defect with severe bone destruction beneath.

Clinical symptoms
Localised tooth mobility and/or severe recession usually in young males less than 20 years of age. It may also present as a localised exophytic swelling (Chapter 5).

Aetiology
Unknown.

Involvement of non-gingival sites
Not with the unifocal lesion, but the condition may become multifocal, with the long bones, cranium and ribs involved.

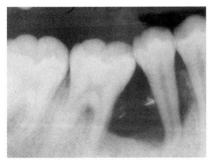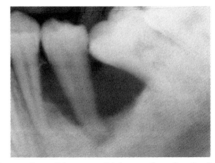

Fig 9-23 Multifocal eosinophilic granulomas in a 14-year-old boy who also had lesions in both femurs. Classical histiocytosis-X (Hand-Schuller-Christian disease).

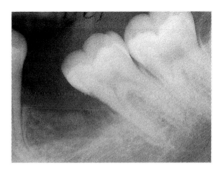

Fig 9-24 The same area as in Fig 9-23 post-chemotherapy and extraction of LL5.

Differential diagnosis
- Localised aggressive (juvenile) periodontitis.
- Hyperparathyroidism (normally females).
- Intra-osseous haemangioma.
- Metastatic tumour (e.g. breast, prostate) – rare.
- Osteosarcoma – rare.

Clinical investigation
Radiographs demonstrate focal osteolytic lesions (Fig 9-23) where local bone destruction may be well or poorly demarcated. Incisional biopsy of the gingiva and underlying connective tissues shows tumour-like collections of histiocytes (Langerhans cells/ tissue macrophages) and eosinophils.

Management options
1. Unifocal eosinophilic granuloma. Medical management will involve bone scanning to eliminate disseminated lesions and either curettage/surgical debridement of the region or local radiotherapy. Fig 9-24 shows the lesions

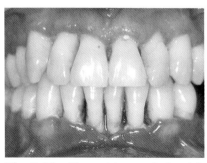

Fig 9-25a Necrotising periodontitis affecting the lower incisors of a patient with HIV disease. Key diagnostic features show loss of gingival contour due to previous papilla ulceration and subsequent papillary blunting. In addition there is ligament and bone loss, and other parts of the mouth are unaffected by the severe attachment loss.

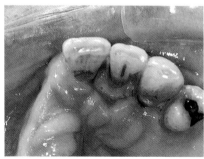

Fig 9-25b More classical NUP, where ulceration is clearly evident, alongside attachment and bone loss UL21 area.

from Fig 9-23 post chemotherapy (and extraction of LL5), following which the prognosis is generally good.

2. Multifocal Eosinophilic Granuloma. Presents with ulcerative mucosal lesions and underlying osteolytic lesions of bone. Multi-focal (often temporal bones) and organ involvement. Lesions of the jaw bones present as for unifocal eosinophilic granuloma and in Hand-Schuller-Christian disease there is:
   - Diabetes insipidus.
   - Skull defects.
   - Exophthalmos.

3. Progressive/Disseminated Histiocytosis (Letterer-Siwe Disease). Tooth mobility due to progressive osteolytic lesions, which may also cause pain. There may be fever, lymphadenopathy, hepato-splenomegaly and a pancytopenia. Usually presenting in infants, it is aggressive and often fatal.

Necrotising Ulcerative Periodontitis (NUP) – see also Chapter 7
Clinical appearance
- Severe recession due to loss of periodontal attachment (Fig 9-25a).
- Flattened gingival margin with loss/blunting and ulceration of the interdental papillae (Fig 9-25b).
- If active, grey sloughing is evident due to interdental tissue necrosis.
- A characteristic anaerobic foetor (halitosis) is evident.

- Significant and immediate bleeding from the gingival margin when probed or spontaneously.
- Regional cervical lymphadenopathy.

Clinical symptoms
- Rapidly receding gums.
- Pain, due to ulceration/bone pain.
- Severe bleeding on brushing.
- Tooth mobility.
- Halitosis/oral malodour.

Aetiology
Classically a fuso-spirochaetal infection with Fusobacterium nucleatum and Treponema vincentii (which invade the tissues) in patients who are immuno-suppressed. Involvement of Prevotella intermedia and Candida species is also reported. Most commonly reported in HIV-infected subjects (prevalence 6.3% – Glick et al 1994) who have a $CD4^+$ count below 400 and a high viral load (>50,000 copies per ml blood). NUP has historically been regarded as an extension of NUG (see Chapple and Gilbert, 2002), involving the periodontal attachment apparatus and alveolar bone, rather than being limited to the gingivae. However, recently it appears to be presenting in young non–HIV-infected patients (mainly females), where the classical risk factors of smoking, poor oral hygiene and stress are present. Additionally a poor diet low in antioxidants and fibre is also evident as a clinical impression.

Involvement of non-gingival sites
Rarely necrotising periodontitis may progress to necrotising stomatitis (Chapple and Hamburger 2000).

Differential diagnosis
- Localised chronic periodontitis (where classical ulceration is absent) with severe recession.
- Trauma from self-mutilation (Fig 9-19).
- Recession due to underlying bone sequestration.
- Use of cocaine or other recreational drugs locally applied to gingivae.

Clinical investigation
- Comprehensive history including:
  - medical history.
  - sexual history.

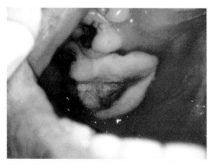

Fig 9-26 Necrotising stomatitis in a patient with AIDS affecting UR 67 area of the palate. The underlying bone was necrotic and teeth non-vital. The brown stain is due to use of chlorhexidine gluconate (0.2%).

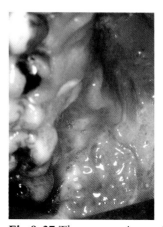

Fig 9-27 The same patient as Fig 9-26, but 18months later with conservative management. The ulceration is shallow, but there is a superficial candidal infection.

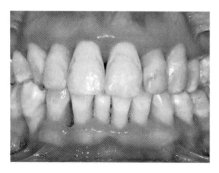

Fig 9-28 Severe recession in a 17-year-old female cocaine user, who presented with gingival ulceration, attachment and bone loss and recession around her lower incisors. Her diet was also poor and low in antioxidants.

  - history of habits (including trauma, drug use, smoking history etc).
  - diet history.
  - past dental history (previous episodes or previous periodontitis).
  - family history.
- Clinical examination:
  - extra-oral (submandibular or cervical lymphadenopathy).
  - intra-oral.
- Presence of foetor oris.
- Microbiology (dark field/phase contrast) will demonstrate spirochaetes.

Management options
- Counselling is essential for the following:
  - smoking.
  - diet.

- stress.
- recreational drug use.
- HIV counselling and testing if deemed necessary from the history.
• Oral hygiene instruction.
• Scaling and root surface debridement with adjunctive systemic metron-idazole 200-400mg TDS seven days.
• Review.
• Referral to genito-urinary medicine if appropriate.

Necrotising Ulcerative Stomatitis (NUS)

NUS is believed to be an extension of NUP involving the oral mucosa and underlying bone in an ulcerative lesion that extends more than 10mm beyond the gingival margin (Fig 9-26). Its behaviour is aggressive leading to necrosis of underlying bone and loss of tooth vitality. There have been reports of oro-nasal fistulae developing (Felix et al 1991).

Recommended treatment is broad surgical excision of the involved area of bone (usually maxilla) back to healthy bleeding bone margins, along with extraction of teeth that are involved in the necrosis and surgical packing of the defect to allow gradual healing by secondary intention, usually under a general anaesthetic. If the patient is a poor anaesthetic or surgical risk, then conservative management should be considered. The patient in Fig 9-26 had lost five stone in weight and was deemed a poor anaesthetic risk, due to the underlying medical condition. Management was therefore conservative, involving oral hygiene instruction, longer-term use of chlorhexidine mouthwash and regular scaling and prophylaxis by domiciliary visits if necessary. The patient survived for 18 months (Fig 9-27) and was pain free and able to eat normally, prior to a fatal infection with PCP (Pneumocystis carinii pneumonia). This case was managed prior to the advent of modern anti-retro viral drugs and HAART (Highly active anti-retro viral therapy).

Drug-Induced Recession

The use of recreational drugs such as cocaine is associated with severe mucositis, ulceration and recession and bone loss when applied to the gingivae. Cocaine is inhaled into the nose as a white crystalline powder, but oral, vaginal and rectal application is also used, as well as intravenous administration. Crack cocaine is smoked. Local application to gingival tissue causes severe inflammation, bleeding and epithelial desquamation, with necrosis of underlying bone and subsequent recession (Fig 9-28).

References

Akerly WB. Prosthodontic treatment of traumatic overlap of the anterior teeth. J Prosthet Dent 1977;38:26-34.
Baxter, AM, Roberts A, Shaw L, Chapple ILC. Localised Scleroderma in a 12-year-old girl presenting as gingival recession. A case report and literature review. Dental Update 2001;28:458-462.

Chapple ILC, Hamburger J. The significance of oral health in HIV disease. J Sexual Transmit Infect 2000;76:236-243.

Chapple ILC, Lumley PJ. Periodontal/endodontic lesions. Dental Update 1999;26:331-341.

Felix DH, Wray D, Smith GLF, et al. Oro-antral fistula: an unusual complication of HIV-associated periodontal disease. Br Dent J 1991;171:61-62.

Glick M, Muzyka BC, Slakin LM et al. Necrotizing ulcerative periodontitis: a marker for immune deterioration and a predictor for the diagnosis of AIDS. J Periodontol 1994;65:393-397.

Tonetti MS, Mombelli A. Early-onset periodontitis. In 1999 International Workshop for a Classification of Periodontal Diseases and Conditions. Annals of Periodontology 1999;4:39-53.

Further Reading

Clerehugh V, Tugnait A, Chapple ILC. Periodontal Management of Children, Adolescents and Young Adults. Chapple ILC (Ed). QuintEssentials of Dental Practice −17, Periodontology-4. London: Quintessence Publishing Co. Ltd, 2004;Chapter 5 pp 79-100.

Heasman PA, Preshaw PM, Robertson P. Successful Periodontal Therapy. A Non-Surgical Approach. Chapple ILC (Ed). QuintEssentials of Dental Practice −16, Periodontology-3. London: Quintessence Publishing Co. Ltd, 2004;Chapter 6 pp83-84.

Noble SN, Kellett M, Chapple ILC. Decision-Making for the Periodontal Team. Chapple ILC (Ed). QuintEssentials of Dental Practice −11, Periodontology-2. London: Quintessence Publishing Co. Ltd, 2004.Chapter 8 pp124 & Chapter 9 142-143.

Watts TLP (Ed). Periodontics in Practice: Science with Humanity. London: Martin Dunitz Ltd, London, 2000;Chapter 4, pp28.

Chapter 10

Generalised Gingival Recession

Aim

To describe the appearance and discuss the aetiology, investigation and periodontal management of systemic diseases that manifest clinically as generalised gingival recession.

Outcome

Having read this chapter, the clinician should be aware of the systemic diseases that may give rise to generalised gingival recession, either directly as a result of the biology of that disease process, or secondary to aggressive periodontal disease, which is a component of that systemic condition. Table 10-1 lists the most common causes of generalised gingival recession, but this chapter will limit discussion to recession associated with underlying systemic diseases. Most of these conditions are uncommon and patients should be referred for specialist management, rather than being managed in general practice.

Background

Gingival recession refers to a situation arising where the gingival margin lies apical to its true position in 'pristine health'. Fig 10-1 illustrates pristine health, which is very rare and quite distinct from 'clinical health'. In clinical health, it is generally accepted that very subtle signs of mild inflammation will be evident at isolated sites and that variations in normal anatomy may result in a dento-alveolar complex with investing periodontal tissues that are not 'classical' in appearance. Fig 10-2 is an example of clinical health, where a midline diastema between the lower incisors provides a non-classical appearance of the interdental papilla and the papilla LL12 has evidence of very mild clinical inflammation.

The detailed anatomy of the dento-gingival complex is discussed in book 1 of this series (Chapple and Gilbert, 2002), and further discussion is not within the remit of this book. However, Fig 10-3 illustrates the normal anatomy of this area and Fig 10-4 provides the reader with a reminder of the contribu-

Table 10-1 **Generalised gingival recession**

Condition	Sub-Category	Nature	Incidence	Manage/Refer
Trauma	Toothbrush Trauma	Facial surfaces	common	manage
		e.g. de-gloving injury	uncommon	manage
	Occlusion	Traumatic class 2 Div II (gingival stripping)	common	manage/refer
Periodontal disease	Untreated		common	manage
	Treated		common	manage
Systematic disease with generalised recession as	Down syndrome	Trisomy chromosome 21	common	manage
	Papillon–Lefevre syndrome (PLS) ± Haim Munk syndrome	Genetic mutation of blood neutrophil gene for enzyme Cathepsin C	uncommon	refer
Manifestation due to	Hypophosphatasia	Genetic defect in gene for enzyme alkaline phosphatase	uncommon	refer
destructive periodontitis	Chronic granulomatous disease (CGD)	Genetic defect – failure of neutrophils to kill bacteria	uncommon	refer
	Chèdiak-Higashi syndrome	Genetic defect of neutrophil function	uncommon	refer
	Ehlers–Danlos syndrome	Genetic defect of collagen metabolism	uncommon	refer

Condition	Sub-Category	Nature	Incidence	Manage/ Refer
	Leukocyte adhesion deficiency (LAD)	Genetic defect of neutrophil affacting ability to adhere	uncommon	refer
	Acatalasia	Genetic defect of catalase production in red blood cells	uncommon	refer
	Infantile genetic agranulocytosis	Severe neutropaenia	uncommon	refer
	Agamma/ hypogammaglobulinaemia	IgG_2 and IgG_4 deficiency	uncommon	refer
	Cohen syndrome	Complex genetic syndrome	uncommon	refer
	Glycogen storage disease	Defect of glygogen metabolism – neutropaenia	uncommon	refer
	DiGeorge syndrome	T-cell defects	uncommon	refer
	Wiskott–Aldrich syndrome	T & B-cell defects	uncommon	refer
	Histiocytosis	Malignant neoplasm of CD-1a cells i.e. Langerhans cells/ histiocytes/ macrophages	uncommon	refer
Systemic disease with recession as manifestation independent of periodontitis	Progressive systemic sclerosis (scleroderma)	Connective tissue disorder	uncommon	refer

185

Condition	Sub-Category	Nature	Incidence	Manage/ Refer
Drug-induced lesions	Cyclophosphamide	Alkylating drug	uncommon	refer
	Methotrexate	Cytotoxic drug	uncommon	refer
	Cocaine	Recreational drug	uncommon	refer
	Bleomycin	Anti–tumour drug	uncommon	refer
	Vincristine/ Vinblastine	Alkaloid drugs	uncommon	refer

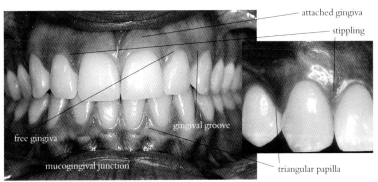

Fig 10-1 An anterior view of 'pristine gingivae', demonstrating applied anatomical features from Fig 10-3.

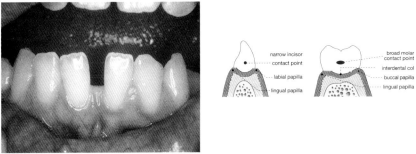

Fig 10-2 Clinical photograph of healthy gingivae, demonstrating the effect of the tooth contact area in dictating interdental papilla shape. The schematic diagrams show the narrow contact point and narrow col between incisors and the broader contact and deeper, more vulnerable col area between molar teeth.

tion of recession to overall periodontal attachment loss. In health, the gingival margin lies on enamel 2-3mm above the position of the terminal cell of the junctional epithelium (JE, Fig 10-3). The JE lies at the cemento-enamel junction (CEJ) and the interval between the terminal cell of the JE and the gingival margin is bordered by JE and sulcular epithelium, which form the soft tissue boundary to the gingival crevice. The crevice can be probed up to a distance of 3mm in health. Clinical attachment loss (CAL) due to periodontitis may arise without recession, by true pocket formation (Fig 10-4), but when the gingival margin migrates to a position apical to the CEJ, recession occurs and contributes, with true pocketing, to overall CAL. The gingival margin may lie at the CEJ, and in this situation there is no recession, but clearly the full clinical crown is exposed and attachment loss has taken place.

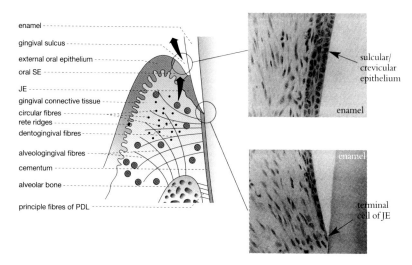

Fig 10-3 A schematic view of the gingivae demonstrating the gingival collagen fibre complexes. The sulcular (SE) and junctional epithelium (JE) are also represented alongside in two photomicrographs demonstrating normal histology. Note how widely spaced the cells are and how they thin out, forming a single 'terminal cell' of the apex of the JE.

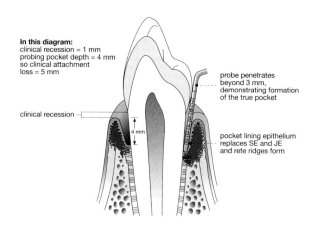

Fig 10-4 Schematic longitudinal section of a premolar and associated periodontal tissues, demonstrating early true pocket formation, detected by probing and recession contributing to overall attachment loss.

Aetiology of Gingival Recession

The most common cause of gingival recession is toothbrush trauma. This classically presents buccally to posterior teeth at the facial surfaces and not the interproximal surfaces. Interproximal recession generally implies CAL due to true periodontitis. Other common causes of generalised recession include:

- untreated periodontal disease (Fig 10-5).
- effects of successful periodontal therapy (Fig 10-6).
- trauma from the occlusion (usually labial stripping of gingivae labial to the lower incisors or palatal to upper incisors in a traumatic class II division 2 malocclusion (see Noble, Kellett and Chapple, 2004).
- physical trauma from an accident (de-gloving injuries from blunt trauma e.g. steering wheel or fist).

This chapter will focus on recession due to periodontal attachment loss that has arisen:

1. secondary to systemic disease where destructive periodontitis is a manifestation of that disease.
2. directly as a manifestation of a systemic disease, even in the absence of significant inflammatory periodontitis (e.g. systemic sclerosis, drug-induced recession).

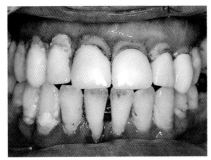

Fig 10-5 Generalised recession due to progressive untreated chronic periodontitis.

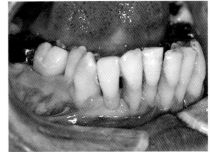

Fig 10-6 Generalised gingival recession following successful periodontal therapy and supportive care. A Maryland bridge has been fabricated to replace LR2, which was lost to periodontal disease.

Systemic Disease with Generalised Recession as Manifestation Due to Destructive Periodontitis

Down Syndrome

Clinical appearance
- Generalised recession upper and lower incisors.
- Severe periodontal destruction and pocketing (Fig 10-7).
- Gingival inflammation.
- Severe radiographic bone loss affecting upper and lower incisors.
- Short roots to lower incisors.
- Tooth mobility.

Clinical symptoms
- Gingival bleeding.
- Tooth mobility (especially lower incisors).
- Impaired eating/function.

Aetiology
Down syndrome, first described by Langdon-Down, is a complex syndrome whose genetic basis is trisomy of chromosome 21. The cause of the periodontal destruction, which is reported to affect between 60-90% of subjects is also complex and thought to involve:
- Poor oral hygiene (especially in institutionalised individuals).
- Defects of PMNL function (chemotaxis, phagocytosis and killing).
- Depressed T-cell induced antigen killing.
- B-lymphocyte receptor defects.
- Abnormal collagen biosynthesis.

Involvement of non-gingival sites
- Characteristic facial appearance (Fig 10-8).
- Learning difficulties.

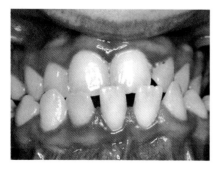

Fig 10-7 Periodontal disease and gingival inflammation in a patient with Down syndrome.

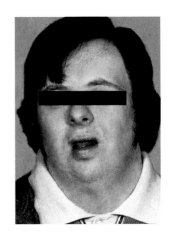

Fig 10-8 The patient from Fig 10-7.

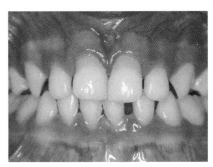

Fig 10-9 A two-year-old Pakistani boy with recession and early mobility of upper and lower deciduous incisors due to Papillon-Lefèvre syndrome (PLS).

- Short stature.
- Cardiac defects (may need antibiotic cover).
- Class III malocclusion.
- Anterior open bite.
- Macroglossia.
- Anterior tooth crowding.

Differential diagnosis
Given the obvious clinical presentation and medical history, no other differential diagnoses are likely.

Clinical investigation
- Standard periodontal investigations.

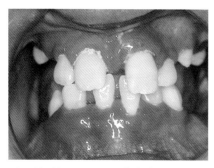

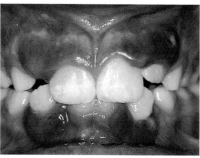

Fig 10-10 Spacing and drifting on the anterior permanent incisors in a seven-year old boy with PLS and severe periodontal disease.

Fig 10-11 Severe gingival inflammation in a six-year old boy, with grade II mobility of the central incisors.

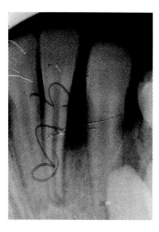

Fig 10-12 Substantial bone loss affecting the permanent dentition of the patient in Fig 10-11.

Management options
- Behavioural management.
- Non-surgical periodontal therapy.
- Rigorous supportive care.
- Cardiological opinion in case antibiotic prophylaxis is needed for invasive procedures.

Papillon-Lefèvre Syndrome
Clinical appearance
Generally presents between the ages of two and seven years with one or more of the following, which affect the deciduous and permanent dentition:
- Generalised recession affecting deciduous incisors (Fig 10-10).

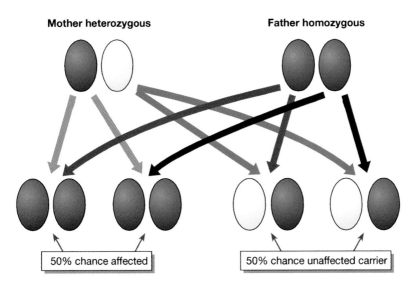

Fig 10-13 The family of the two-year old boy with PLS (Fig 10-9) demonstrating the Mendelian pattern of autosomal recessive inheritance of the condition.

- Premature tooth mobility.
- Spacing and drifting of anterior teeth (Fig 10-10).
- Severe generalised gingival inflammation (Fig 10-11).
- Severe periodontal destruction radiographically (Fig 10-12).
- Radiographic bone loss where apices of permanent teeth are not yet fully formed.

Patients generally progress to total tooth loss by 20 years of age.

Clinical symptoms
- Gingival recession.
- Tooth mobility.
- Gingival bleeding.
- Tooth spacing.
- Recurrent abscesses/infection.

Aetiology
Papillon-Lefèvre syndrome (PLS) is an inherited autosomal recessive disorder, characterised by a strong family history of consanguinity (Fig 10-13). It has a prevalence of one in four million, most common in Indo-Pakistani

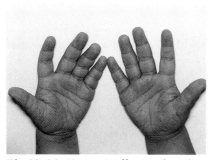

Fig 10-14a Keratosis affecting the palms of the hands of a two-year-old boy with Papillon Lefevre syndrome (PLS). The gene mutation was a common mutation (R272P).

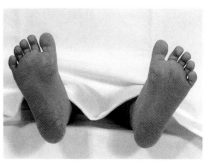

Fig 10-14b Keratosis affecting the soles of the feet of the two-year old boy in Fig 10-14a.

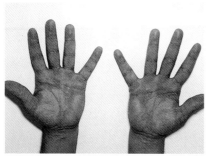

Fig 10-15a Keratosis affecting the palms of the hands of the father of the two-year old boy with PLS in Fig 10-14a.

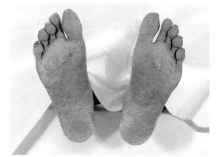

Fig 10-15b Keratosis affecting the soles of the feet in the patient in Fig 10-15a.

children, and classical signs usually appear between two and four years of age. It arises from a gene defect, recently mapped to the long arm of chromosome 11 (11q) and results in the loss of function of an important neutrophil (PMNL) enzyme called Cathepsin-C. Cathepsin-C is a lysosomal enzyme found in the primary granules of PMNLs that is important in bacterial destruction and is expressed in the skin of the feet and hands, as well as lung, kidney and placenta.

Involvement of non-gingival sites
- Classical palmar-plantar keratoderma (hyperkeraotsis of the palms of the hands and soles of the feet (Fig 10-14 and 10-15).

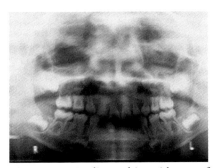

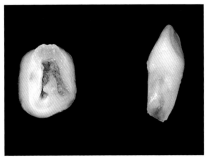

Fig 10-16a Radiographic evidence of premature deciduous tooth loss in a five-year-old boy with hypophosphatasia.

Fig 10-16b Enlarged pulp chambers of teeth that spontaneously exfoliated from the patient in Fig 10-16a.

- Intracranial calcifications are occasionally reported.
- Another rare syndrome Haim Munk syndrome (HMS), presents with similar features, but has only been reported in two families at the time of going to press. HMS was first reported in a Jewish sect from Cochin, India and patients present with the same features as in PLS, but also suffer from:
  - Recurrent pyogenic skin infections.
  - Arachnodactyly (long, slender fingers).
  - Acro-osteolysis (osteolysis of distal phalanges).
  - Onychogryphosis (curved thickening of nails).
  - Pes planus (flat feet/fallen arches of the feet).

The patient in Fig 10-10 first presented with recurrent skin infections, but the diagnosis was not made until he developed tooth mobility and was seen by the author, when PLS was diagnosed following careful history taking, clinical examination and genetic testing. The relationship between PLS and HMS is becoming clearer and they appear to be either allelic variants (Hart et al, 2000), i.e. different mutations in the same gene, although the same mutation has been reported in PLS as in HMS. Alternatively, it is also possible that HMS is a variant of PLS, arising following co-inheritance of a further, yet to be identified gene mutation in the vicinity of the CTSC gene locus. This has been demonstrated previously for co-inheritance of PLS with albinism (Hewitt et al, 2004). To date 45 different mutations have been described in the Cathepsin C gene, including a symptom free mutation (Allende et al, 2000).

Differential diagnosis
- Hypophosphatasia (see later in chapter).
- Chronic granulomatous disease (CGD) – failure of the respiratory burst within PMNLs and therefore failure of oxygen radicals to destroy bacteria. However, usually severe gingival inflammation and ulceration/recession are reported but not an aggressive periodontitis (see Clerehugh, Tugnait and Chapple, 2004).
- Chèdiak-Higashi syndrome (see later in chapter).
- Ehlers-Danlos syndrome (see later in chapter).
- Leukocyte adhesion deficiency (LAD – see later in chapter).
- Acatalasia – (see later in chapter).
- Infantile genetic agranulocytosis (see later in chapter).
- Cohen syndrome – autosomal recessive, characterised by extensive alveolar bone loss, neutropenia, learning difficulties, motor function defects, dysmorphia, obesity.
- Glycogen storage disease – series of five conditions involving impairment/inability to metabolise glygogen. In type 1B (autosomal recessive) patients have neutropaenia, defective PNML function and periodontal disease.
- DiGeorge syndrome – defects of T-lymphocyte function caused by a gene deletion on chromosome 22q (q = long arm of chromosome; p = short arm).
- Wiskott-Aldrich syndrome – X-linked T and B-cell immune deficiency.
- Histiocytosis – usually localised recession defects (see chapter 10).

Clinical investigation
- PLS is a diagnosis made following collection of a family history and clinical findings.
- Cranial radiographs may reveal calcifications of the cerebral membranes.
- Genetic testing is not available routinely.

Management options
Genetic counselling for parents is essential (pre-natal mutation analysis is available). Management is very difficult because most evidence is based on case reports, or at best case series and most reports have demonstrated poor efficacy of both surgical and non-surgical therapy. However, strict plaque control can slow down the progression of the disease and current thinking is that success rates may be improved by:
- Early extraction of deciduous dentition to provide a period of edentulousness, and eliminate pathogens from the mouth.

- Scaling and root surface debridement of permanent teeth in conjunction with systemic antibiotics.
- Bi-weekly professional prophylaxis and repeated mechanical therapy after identification of Actinobacillus actinomycetemcomitans (Aa).
- Systemic retinoid therapy - Acitretin has been shown to correct defective CD3-induced human T-lymphocyte activation in vitro in PLS patients. Retinoids may also regulate Cathepsin C gene expression, but should be prescribed by specialists due to their side effects.

The case in Fig 10-9 was managed by:
1. Full mouth scaling and prophylaxis whilst taking systemic amoxicillin and metronidazole.
2. Treatment of his dentate mother (as above) despite the absence of periodontal disease, in order to eliminate Aa. The father was edentulous and therefore deemed unlikely to possess the relevant pathogens.
3. Restricted close contact with grandparents who lived in the family home.
4. Four- to six- weekly recalls for full mouth prophylaxis.

By the age of four the patient still had a full deciduous dentition, whereas in most patients bone loss is so rapid that total deciduous tooth loss by four years of age is common. At 4.5 years the lower right deciduous incisor was electively extracted due to severe mobility and the full course of debridement repeated with systemic Augmentin (Co-amoxiclav). At the time of this book going to press, the child was 5.5 years old and his periodontal condition was starting to deteriorate, leading to consideration of a deciduous dentition clearance and retinoid therapy.

Hypophosphatasia
Clinical appearance
- Severe recession (often localised to incisors) in a child or young adult (deciduous or permanent dentition).
- Severe tooth mobility.
- Often minimal gingival inflammation.
- Premature deciduous tooth loss.
- Premature eruption of permanent successors.
- Radiographic bone loss especially anterior teeth, largely horizontal.
- Enlarged dental pulp chambers to teeth radiologically.

Clinical symptoms
- Early deciduous tooth loss.

- Teeth exfoliate with intact roots (i.e. no/minimal resorption).
- Tooth mobility.

Aetiology
Hypophosphatasia has five subtypes and is a rare inherited defect in the enzyme alkaline phosphatase (ALP). It affects 1:100,000 and evidence exists for allelic forms, one autosomal dominant (presenting with milder features) and one autosomal recessive (severe phenotype). Gene mutations can give rise to:

1. Perinatal (or lethal) hypophosphatasia – where infants live only a few days (rachitic chest leads to respiratory failure).
2. Infantile hypophosphatasia - First six months of life, presents with systemic manifestations (wide fontanelles, blue sclera, flail chest, poor feeding/weight gain).
3. Childhood hypophosphatasia (Fig 10-16a and b).
- Premature deciduous tooth loss.
- Cementum hypoplasia or aplasia (cementum does not form on roots).
- Disuse atrophy of alveolus as no connection exists for periodontal ligament fibres at the root surface due to lack of cementum.
- Wide open cranial fontanelles may be evident (anterior and posterior).
- Skull has a 'beaten copper' appearance.
- Proptosis (bulging eyes) may be evident due to premature fusion of cranial sutures.
4. Adult hypophosphatasia – has a mild phenotype and often presents in middle age. There may be a history of early deciduous tooth loss and the anterior six maxillary and mandibular incisors tend to be affected.
5. Pseudohypophosphatasia – or odontohypophosphatasia - is very mild and tends to be localised to the lower anterior deciduous teeth.

Involvement of non-gingival sites
This varies according to the type of hypophosphatasia. For detailed review see Chapple et al, 1993.

Differential diagnosis
- PLS
- Chèdiak-Higashi syndrome.
- Ehlers-Danlos syndrome.
- Leukocyte adhesion deficiency.
- Acatalasia.

Clinical investigation
Diagnosis involves:
- Radiology.
- Clinical biochemistry. Due to the deficiency of the liver/bone/kidney iso-enzyme of ALP, substrates normally metabolised by ALP appear raised. In addition to low levels of ALP in serum (ensure normal range is used for children or adults, as appropriate), raised levels of:
  - Pyridoxal-5-phosphate (PLP or vitamin B6) are found in serum
  - Phosphoethanolamine in 24-hour urine samples.

Management options
Currently, management options include:
- Genetic counselling
- Intensive non-surgical periodontal therapy.

Chronic Granulomatous Disease (CGD)
This is a rare condition that does not normally cause significant recession and therefore discussion will be brief. CGD is reported in autosomal and X-linked recessive forms. The respiratory burst that creates the oxygen radical superoxide (see Chapple and Gilbert, 2002) and subsequently hydrogen peroxide and other reactive oxygen species within PMNL's fails. Therefore, bacteria are phagocytosed by PMNLs and released in a viable state rather than being destroyed. Unsurprisingly, sufferers have severely compromised infection control mechanisms, rendering them susceptible to osteomyelitis and pneumonia. Reported periodontal manifestations seem to be limited to severe gingival inflammation and ulceration, which may lead to recession, rather than periodontal destruction.

Chèdiak-Higashi Syndrome
Clinical appearance
- Severe gingival inflammation.
- Suppurative periodontitis with tooth mobility and generalised recession.
- Early deciduous tooth loss.
- Severe periodontal bone loss.

Clinical symptoms
- Bleeding gums.
- Early tooth loss.
- Tooth mobility.

Aetiology
A rare autosomal recessive condition, Chèdiak–Higashi syndrome is regarded as an inherited disorder of the blood/lymphoreticular system. It largely affects PMNL and monocyte function. Defects include:
• Impaired chemotaxis.
• Defective bacterial killing (phagolysosome formation is impaired – see Chapple and Gilbert, 2002).
• Defective degranulation and release of oxygen radicals.
• Hyper-responsive phagocytosis but ineffective killing.

Involvement of non-gingival sites
• Oral ulceration.
• High susceptibility to bacterial infections.

Differential diagnosis
• PLS.
• Hypophosphatasia.
• Ehlers–Danlos syndrome.
• Leukocyte adhesion deficiency.
• Acatalasia.

Clinical investigation
• Careful history of bacterial infections
• Immunological investigations of neutrophil chemotaxis, adhesion and killing.

Management options
A variety of drug regimes have been described, starting with milder therapies such as vitamin-C supplementation, to the use of cytotoxic drugs (e.g. methotrexate, vincristine), which are themselves associated with gingival ulceration and recession. The use of corticosteroids has also been advocated.

Ehlers–Danlos Syndrome
Clinical appearance
• Severe generalised recession.
• Fragile gingival tissues prone to excessive bleeding and bruising.
• Generalised aggressive periodontal pocketing and bone loss.

Clinical symptoms
• Gum recession.
• Generalised profuse gingival bleeding.

- Tooth mobility.
- Early tooth loss.

Aetiology
This is a rare genetic syndrome with varying inheritance according to the subtype diagnosed. It involves defects of collagen synthesis and 10 subtypes are described, with aggressive periodontal destruction associated with type IV (autosomal recessive or dominant), type VIII (autosomal recessive or dominant) and type IX (X-linked).

Involvement of non-gingival sites
- Excessive joint mobility (subluxation of temporomandibular joints is reported).
- Skin hyperextensibility (Fig 10-17).
- Excessive bruising due to blood vessel fragility.
- Post-extraction haemorrhage.
- Poor/delayed healing.
- Cardiac valve involvement.

Differential diagnosis
- PLS.
- Hypophosphatasia.
- Chèdiak-Higashi syndrome.
- Leukocyte adhesion deficiency.
- Acatalasia.

Clinical investigation
- History (including family history).
- Examination for signs of skin hyperextensibility.

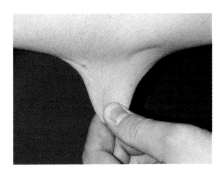

Fig 10-17 Skin hyperextensibility in Ehlers-Danlos syndrom.

- Laboratory investigations of pro-collagen and collagen production (immunohistochemistry) from biopsy samples.
- Genetic testing.

Management options
Very little data is available and referral recommended due to the complications associated with tissue fragility and excessive haemorrhage.

Leukocyte Adhesion Deficiency (LAD)
Clinical appearance
- Severe generalised recession.
- Deciduous tooth loss almost immediately on eruption.
- Fiery red gingivae.
- Profuse gingival bleeding.

Clinical symptoms
- Gingival bleeding.
- Early tooth loss.
- Recurrent infections.

Aetiology
LAD is a rare condition inherited in an autosomal recessive manner (reviewed by Kinane 1999). They involve defects in 3 key leukocyte cell surface receptors called β–integrins (see Chapple and Gilbert 2002) that have important functions including binding complement and helping PMNL's enter the tissues from within blood vessels (Table 10-2). Such defects give rise to significant PMNL-binding problems and hence dramatically affect the patient's ability to fight infection. The LADs are heterogeneous conditions and patients with severe LAD (<0.3% of receptors) do not survive long after birth, whereas patients with milder phenotypes survive to adulthood but suffer various illnesses, including a severe form of pre–pubertal periodontitis.

Involvement of non-gingival sites
- Papules and nodules affecting the mucosa of the cheeks are reported
- Recurrent and multiple infections.

Differential diagnosis
- PLS.
- Hypophosphatasia.
- Ehlers-Danlos syndrome.

Table 10-2 **White blood cell receptors relevant to leukocyte adhesion deficiency (LAD), their names and codes**

Receptor	Cells that Express	Other Names	Cluster of differentiation (CD) marker designation
CR3 (binds complement component C3)	Monocytes PMNL NK cells	Mac-1	CD 11b (α-chain of CR3)
CR4 (binds complement component C3)	PMNL Monocytes NK cells	P150,95	CD 11c (α-chain of CR4)
LFA-1 (Leucocyte function antigen-1)	Monocytes Macrophages PMNL Lymphocytes		CD 11a (α-chain of LFA-1)

- Chèdiak–Higashi syndrome.
- Acatalasia.

Clinical investigation
- Studies of cell surface receptor defects.

Management options
These are limited to medical referral and maintaining periodontal care of the highest standard.

Acatalasia
Acatalasia is a rare inherited autosomal recessive condition in which the key intracellular antioxidant enzyme catalase is deficient. Catalase is present mainly in red blood cells but also PMNLs and removes excess hydrogen peroxide (H_2O_2) before it causes damage to vital cell structures through oxidation reactions and upregulation of pro-inflammatory cytokine release by nuclear transcription factors like NFκB (equation 1).

$$2H_2O_2 \xrightarrow{\text{catalase}} 2H_2O + O_2 \qquad \text{– equation 1}$$

When PMNLs are stimulated by periodontal pathogens or their products, they produce reactive oxygen species (ROS) like H_2O_2 which are important in microbial destruction. However, excessive ROS production, if not neutralised by key antioxidants is now known to be a major cause of 'collateral' periodontal tissue damage (Chapple, 1997; Brock et al, 2004). Deficiency in catalase facilitates such destructive processes and is associated with severe periodontal destruction, necrosis and ulceration. Interestingly, the role of catalase in the extracellular environment is performed by a very important enzyme, glutathione peroxidase (GSH-Px), which is largely selenium-dependent and reduces (H_2O_2) whilst oxidising reduced glutathione (GSH) to its oxidised form (GSSG).

$$2GSH + H_2O_2 \xrightarrow{\text{GSH-Px}} GSSG + 2H_2O \qquad \text{–equation 2}$$

Recently, we have reported a deficiency in GSH levels in chronic periodontitis subjects (Chapple et al, 2002).

Infantile Genetic Agranulocytosis
This is a rare autosomal recessive disorder that involves a severe neutropenia and is characterised by an aggressive periodontitis, recession and bone loss.

Cohen Syndrome

Cohen syndrome is a rare inherited autosomal recessive condition, characterised by:

- Extensive alveolar bone loss (associated with a neutropenia).
- Learning difficulties.
- Motor function defects.
- Obesity.
- Dysmorphia.

Glycogen Storage Disease

The glycogen storage diseases are a series of five conditions characterised by an inability to metabolise or break down glycogen. Type 1B is autosomal recessive and patients are neutropaenic and demonstrate defective neutrophil function, with associated periodontal disease.

DiGeorge Syndrome

This is a rare primary immune deficiency disease, largely affecting T-lymphocyte function, the cause being a gene deletion from the long arm of chromosome 22. There are various facial abnormalities reported, including cleft palate and an aggressive form of periodontitis has been described in children.

Wiskott-Aldrich Syndrome

Wiscott-Aldrich syndrome is an X-linked immune deficiency involving a deficiency of T and B-cells and thrombocytopaenia.

Histiocytosis X

Histiocytosis X is discussed in Chapter 9.

Systemic Disease with Generalised Recession as Manifestation Independent of Periodontitis

Progressive Systemic Sclerosis (Scleroderma)

Clinical appearance

- Generalised gingival recession (Fig 10-18).
- Tooth mobility.
- Radiographic widening of the periodontal ligament.
- Normal periodontal attachment level and sulcus depth unless coincidental periodontitis is also present, which has a higher reported frequency in scleroderma.

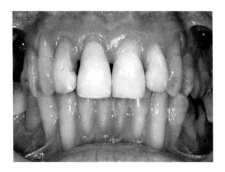

Fig 10-18 Generalised gingival recession in a patient with progressive systemic sclerosis.

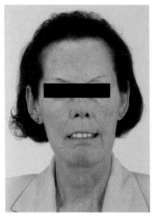

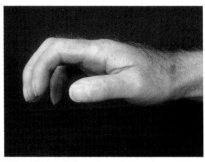

Fig 10-20 Sclerodactyly in the patient shown in Fig 10-18.

Fig 10-19 Tightening of the skin and mask-like facial appearance in the same patient as Fig 10-18.

Clinical symptoms
- Gum recession.
- Sensitivity.
- Tooth mobility.

Involvement of non-gingival sites
- Tight inflexible skin due to fibrosis (mask-like face – Fig 10-19).
- Microstomia (small opening to mouth).
- Xerostomia (secondary Sjögren's syndrome).
- Dysphagia (due to oesophageal stricture).
- Scarring and contracture of fingers (sclerdactyly – Fig 10-20).
- Raynaud's syndrome (numbness/cyanosis of fingers and toes when cold due to vasospasm).

206

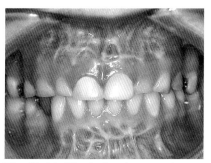

Fig 10-21 Gingival and mucosal scarring.

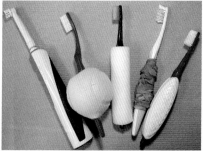

Fig 10-22 A toothbrush handle modified using circular foam to make gripping the handle easier in patients with sclerdactyly.

- Telangectasia.
- Osteolytic lesions within skeletal bone. Mandibular changes involve remodelling or loss of the coronoid process and angle of the mandible.
- Visceral involvement.

Differential diagnosis
- Limited systemic sclerosis (formerly known as CREST – Calcinosis, Raynauds, Esophagitis, Sclerdactyly, Telangectasia).
- Progressive systemic sclerosis.
- Submucous fibrosis.
- Associated with Thibierge-Weissenach syndrome (exrtensive subcutaneous calcifications).

Aetiology
Scleroderma is a rare connective tissue disorder characterised by progressive collagen deposition beneath mucosal and skin surfaces. Gingival and mucosal scarring can appear dramatic (Fig 10–21). Visceral involvement can involve the lungs, heart and kidneys and such patients have a poor prognosis

Clinical investigation
- Serology may identify anti–centromere and/or anti-Scl-70 antibodies. The former can be seen in up to 70% of patients with limited systemic sclerosis and in rather fewer patients with progressive systemic sclerosis.
- Biopsy.

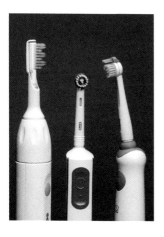

Fig 10-23 Power toothbrushes have larger handles and reduce the necessity for dexterity. Three brushes are shown from an array of many. Sonic powered brushes offer the advantage for these patients of not needing to apply force to or manipulate the bristles.

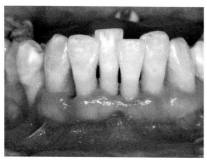

Fig 10-24 Severe recession and bone destruction (similar to necrotising periodontitis) in a 17-year-old female who used cocaine orally.

Management options
• Manage periodontal tissues as for any other patient, but with more regular supportive care.
• It may be necessary to adapt toothbrush handles where sclerodactyly is evident (Fig-10-22) and use smaller toothbrush heads in the presence of microstomia. Modern power toothbrushes may be valuable in such cases (Fig 10-23).

Drug-Induced Gingival Recession
Cytotoxic chemotherapy drugs
Cytotoxic drugs such as cyclophosphamide and methotrexate work by targeting tumour cells with a high rate of division. Gingival epithelium has a naturally high turnover rate (especially JE) and is therefore prone to mucositis, ulceration and recession.

Recreational drugs

Some individuals use cocaine as an oral application, by rubbing the powder into the gingivae. Cocaine has a powerful vasoconstrictive effect and this leads to ulceration, recession and sometimes severe bone resorption, providing an appearance similar to necrotising periodontitis (Fig 10-24).

Cytotoxic antimicrobials

Cytotoxic antimicrobials such as bleomycin, vincristine and vinblastine produce similar affects to cyclophosphamide and methotrexate.

Further Reading

Allende LM, Garcia-Pèrez MA, Moreno A et al. Cathepsin C gene: first compound heterozygous patient with Papillon-Lefèvre syndrome and a novel symptomless mutation. Human Mutation 2000;399:1-6.

Brock G, Matthews JB, Butterworth C J, Chapple ILC. Local and systemic antioxidant capacity in periodontal health. J Clin Periodontol 2004;31:15-21.

Chapple ILC. Hypophosphatasia: dental aspects and mode of inheritance. Journal of Clinical Periodontology 1993;20:615-622.

Chapple ILC. Reactive oxygen species and antioxidants in inflammatory diseases. J Clin Periodontol 1997;24:287-296.

Chapple ILC, Gilbert AD. Understanding Periodontal Diseases: Assessment and Diagnostic Procedures and Practice. Chapple ILC (Ed). QuintEssentials of Dental Practice −1, Periodontology-1. London: Quintessence Publishing Co. Ltd, 2002;Chapter 1 pp3-16.

Chapple ILC, Brock G, Eftimiadi C, Matthews JB. Glutathione in gingival crevicular fluid and its relation to local antioxidant capacity in periodontal health and disease. J Clin Pathol: Molec Pathol 2002, 78:55, 367-373.

Clerehugh V, Tugnait A, Chapple ILC. Periodontal Management of Children, Adolescents and Young Adults. 2004. Chapple ILC (Ed). QuintEssentials of Dental Practice −17, Periodontology-4, London: Quintessence Publishing Co. Ltd, 2004. Chapter 10 pp131-149.

Hart TC, Hart PC, Michalec MD et al. Haim-Munk syndrome and Papillon-Lefèvre syndrome are allelic mutations in Cathepsin C. J Med Genet 2000;37:88-94.

Hewitt C, Wu CL, Hattab FN et al. Coinheritance of two rare genodermatoses (Papillon- Lefèvre syndrome and oculocutaneous albinism type 1) in two families: a genetic study. Br J Dermatol 2004;151:1261-1265.

Kinane DF. Blood and lymphoreticular disorders. Periodontol 2000 1999;21:84-93.

Seymour RA, Heasman PH (Eds). Drugs Diseases and the Periodontium. Oxford: Oxford Medical Publications, 1992.

Chapter 11

Miscellaneous Lesions

Aim

This chapter aims to outline the non plaque-induced periodontal lesions and manifestations of systemic diseases that do not readily fall under the descriptive headings used in the previous 10 chapters. These lesions present primarily as incidental or intentional radiological findings, as gingival bleeding that is inconsistent with local irritants, as para-gingival swellings or annular lesions.

Outcome

At the end of this chapter the reader should have a clear insight into the nature, diagnosis and management of lesions that are discussed therein.

Introduction

Table 11-1 summarises the non-radiological lesions to be discussed. Tables 11-2 to 11-4 list those lesions normally detected radiologically and consistent with the general approach taken within this text, categorised by radiological appearance. The approach taken is similar to that of Langlais, Langeland and Nortjé in Diagnostic Imaging of the Jaws, which is recommended for further reading. Radiological features of periodontitis are not discussed, and those lesions of the soft tissues that can appear on radiographic films are also beyond the scope of this chapter. Only those lesions and conditions likely to present to the periodontal clinician rather than the radiologist will be discussed briefly.

Uncontrolled/Unexplained Gingival Bleeding

When patients present with gingival bleeding that is not consistent with levels of plaque or inflammation, underlying systemic disease should be suspected and appropriate investigations undertaken.

Myelodysplasia

The myelodysplastic syndromes (MDS) are rare haematological disorders of the myeloid cell lineages. They have an incidence of 4:100,000, are hetero-

Table 11-1 Miscellaneous lesions presenting in and around the periodontal tissues

Category	Condition	Sub–Classification	Discussed or Refer Reader
Uncontrolled/un–explained gingival bleeding	Myelodysplasia	Primary Secondary	discussed discussed
	Clotting factor deficiencies	Factor VIII Factor IX	discussed discussed
	Idiopathic thrombocytopenic purpura (ITP)		discussed
	Platelet pool storage disease		discussed
	Acute leukaemia		discussed
	Chronic leukaemia		discussed
	Thrombocytopaenia	Secondary to liver disease Drug–induced HIV–associated Benign familial thrombocytopaenia	discussed discussed discussed discussed
	Aplastic anaemia		discussed
	Thrombasthenia		discussed
	Patients on warfarin		discussed

Category	Condition	Sub-Classification	Discussed or Refer Reader
Para-gingival swellings	Osteomas		discussed
	Gardner's syndrome		discussed
	Mandibular/maxillary tori		discussed
Annular lesions	Erythema migrans		discussed
	Erythema multiforme	Stevens Johnson syndrome	discussed

Table 11-2 **Radiological lesions or conditions involving or associated with the roots**

Radiological Categorisation	Condition	Sub-group	Discussed or Refer Reader
Root resorption	Internal root resorption		reader referred
	External root resorption	Cervical	discussed
		Infra-cervical	
	Inter- and peri-radicular radiolucencies	Scleroderma (systemic sclerosis)	discussed
	Periapical cemental dysplasia		discussed
	Lateral developmental periodontal cyst (Botyroid cyst)		discussed
	Lateral inflammatory periodontal cyst		discussed
	Gingival cyst		discussed
	Incisive canal cyst		discussed
	Solitary bone cyst		reader referred
	Median mandibular cyst		reader referred
	Squamous odontogenic tumour		discussed
	Ameloblastoma	Classical	discussed
		Unicystic	
		Peripheral	
		Malignant	
	Ameloblastic fibroma		discussed

Radiological Categorisation	Condition	Sub-group	Discussed or Refer Reader
	Histiocytosis-X	Unifocal (solitary eosinophilic granuloma)	discussed
Inter- and peri-radicular radiopacities	Periapical osteosclerosis (sclerosing osteitis)		discussed
	Condensing osteitis		discussed
	Hypercementosis		discussed
	Cementomas	Cementoblastoma	discussed
		Periapical cemental dysplasia	discussed
		Gigantiform cementoma	discussed
	Cementicles		discussed
	Ossifying fibroma		discussed

Table 11–3 **Radiolucent lesions**

Radiological Categorisation	Condition	Sub-group	Discussed or Refer Reader
Well circumscribed radiolucencies	Odontogenic keratocyst		discussed
	Inflammatory cysts	Periapical	discussed
		Peri–implant	discussed
	Neural sheath tumours	Neurilemmoma	discussed
		Schwannoma	discussed
		Neurofibroma	discussed
		Neurofibromatosis	discussed
Multi-locular radiolucencies	Odontogenic keratocyst and Gorlin–Goltz syndrome		discussed
	Botyroid cyst (lateral developmental periodontal cyst)		discussed
	Ameloblastoma	Polycystic	discussed
		Malignant	discussed
	Odontogenic myxoma		discussed
	Giant cell tumour of bone (central giant cell granuloma)		discussed
	Arterio-venous malformation		
	Aneurysmal bone cyst		discussed
	Central haemangioma		discussed
	Sturge Weber syndrome	Arterio-venous malformations	reader referred discussed

Radiological Categorisation	Condition	Sub-group	Discussed or Refer Reader
	Cherubism		discussed
	Odontogenic fibroma		reader referred
	Ossifying fibroma	Calcifying/ossifying fibrous epulis	discussed
Poorly defined radiolucent lesions	Osteomyelitis	Sterile	discussed
	Osteoradionecrosis	Septic	discussed
	Intraosseous carcinoma		discussed
	(Epidermoid carcinoma) Gingival carcinoma	Squamous cell	discussed
		Cuniculatum	discussed
	Mucoepidermoid carcinoma		reader referred
	Clear cell carcinoma		reader referred
	Ameloblastic carcinoma		discussed
	Metastatic tumour	Adenocarcinoma of lung	reader referred
		Prostate carcinoma	reader referred
		Breast carcinoma	reader referred
		Renal carcinoma	reader referred
		Melanoma	reader referred

Radiological Categorisation	Condition	Sub-group	Discussed or Refer Reader
	Fibrosarcoma		reader referred
	Ewings sarcoma		reader referred
Radiolucent lesions as presentations of disseminated disease	Histiocytosis-X	Progressive (disseminated or Letterer-Siwe disease)	discussed
		Multifocal (Hand-Schuller-Christian syndrome)	discussed
	Multiple myleoma		discussed
	Non-Hodgkins lymphoma		discussed
	Burkitt's lymphoma		reader referred
	Leukaemia		discussed
Generalised radiolucencies	Hypophosphatasia	Neonatal (Lethal)	discussed
		Infantile	discussed
		Childhood	discussed
		Adult	discussed
		Pseudo-hypophosphatasia (Odontohypophosphatasia)	discussed
	Hyperparathyroidism	Brown tumours	discussed
	Sickle cell anaemia		discussed
	β-thalassaemia		reader referred

Radiological Categorisation	Condition	Sub-group	Discussed or Refer Reader
Radiolucent lesions with radiopacities	Periapical cemental dysplasia		discussed
	Calcifying odontogenic cyst		discussed
	Calcifying epithelial odontogenic tumour		discussed
	Adenomatoid odontogenic tumour		discussed
	Ameloblastic fibroadenoma		reader referred
	Odontomes	Compound	discussed
		Complex	discussed

Table 11-4 **Radio-opaque lesions**

Radiological Categorisation	Condition	Sub-group	Discussed or Refer Reader
Focal radio-opacities	Garrè's osteomyelitis		reader referred
	Hyperostosis		reader referred
	Osteoma		discussed
	Osteoblastoma		reader referred
	Osteoclastoma		reader referred
	Osteosarcoma		discussed
	Osteogenic sacroma		reader referred
	Chondroma		reader referred
	Chondroblastoma		reader referred
	Chondrosarcoma		reader referred
Generalised radiopacities	Gardner's syndrome		discussed
	Osseous dysplasia		reader referred
	Sclerosing osteomyelitis		discussed
	Fibrous dysplasia		discussed
	Albright's syndrome		discussed
	Paget's disease		discussed
	Osteopetrosis	Albers-Schönberg disease	discussed
	Hyperostosis		discussed

geneic in nature and thought to be part of the same spectrum of disorders that give rise to acute myeloid leukaemia (AML). Previously called 'pre-leukaemia', MDS has been diagnosed following persistent herpes labialis, severe oral mucosal ulceration and unexplained or spontaneous gingival bleeding, which was inconsistent with plaque levels (Chapple et al, 1999). The incidence of MDS appears to be increasing, and due to the high mortality rates associated with this group of disorders, it is important that the dental surgeon, who may be the first person to whom patients with MDS present, is aware of this group of disorders. Presentation is normally in patients over 60 years of age.

Clotting Factor Deficiencies
Clotting factor deficiencies that may give rise to excessive gingival bleeding include:
- Von-Willebrand Factor deficiency (important for platelet adhesion).
- Factor II.
- Factor VII.
- Factor VIII (haemophilia). Many haemophiliacs now self-manage by injection of recombinant factor VIII.
- Factor IX (congenital factor IX disease, also called Christmas disease or haemophilia B).
- Factor X.
- Factor XII deficiency (Hageman factor).

Idiopathic Thrombocytopenic Purpura (ITP)
ITP is a chronic autoimmune condition of insidious onset without any identifiable or associated illness. It is a chronic condition that typically affects young and middle aged adults, with a female: male ratio of 3:1. In 30% of adults it is persistent and appears resistant to most forms of treatment. The pathogenesis involves increased platelet destruction by autoantibodies to platelet membrane antigens (glycoprotein 11b/111a).

Platelet Pool Storage Disease
This is a mild congenital bleeding disorder, generally managed by Desmopressin acetate (DDAVP) medication. It is associated with:
- Glanzmann's thrombasthenia – a condition caused by lack of a protein required for platelet aggregation, bleeding might be severe.
- Bernard-Soulier syndrome – a congenital disorder where platelets lack receptors to adhere to vessel walls. Bleeding may also be severe with this disorder.

Acute Leukaemia
This is discussed in Chapter 8.

Chronic Leukaemia
See Chapter 8.

Thrombocytopaenia
Thrombocytopaenia is by definition a platelet deficiency, the defining level being <150,000 platelets per ml of blood. In clinical terms, control of haemorrhage does not normally become a problem in non-surgical periodontal

therapy unless platelet levels fall below 60,000 per ml. There may be many underlying causes of thrombocytopaenia and these include:
- Advanced liver disease.
- HIV-associated thrombocytopaenia.
- Secondary to immunosuppressant and cytotoxic drugs.
- Idiopathic thrombocytopaenic purpura (ITP).
- Platelet pool storage disease.
- Other auto-immune diseases.
- Wiskott-Aldrich syndrome.

Aplastic Anaemia
This is a rare condition that is associated with reduced haemopoetic tissue and a pancytopaenia. Gingival bleeding and advanced periodontal bone loss have been reported.

Thrombasthenia
See Glanzmann's thrombasthenia above.

Patients on Warfarin
Warfarin is the most commonly employed anticoagulant used in patients with a history of:
- Cerebro-vascular accident (stroke).
- Myocardial infarction.
- Thyrotoxicosis with associated cardiac arrhythmias.

Warfarin is a competitive antagonist of vitamin K, which is required for the production in the liver of Factors II, VII, IX and X. These factors are utilised in the coagulation cascade. Warfarin affects the prothrombin time (a measure of the extrinsic coagulation pathway), which is measured in a standardised way as the International Normalised Ratio (INR). An INR of 1.0 is normal, but an increasing ratio is associated with reduced coagulation. A growing body of opinion suggests that provided the INR is ≤ 4 and, local haemostatic measures are employed, periodontal and minor oral surgical procedures can be carried out with minimal post-operative haemorrhage. It is, therefore, less likely that warfarin doses may need to be adjusted in such patients. However, certain drugs may potentiate the action of warfarin and these include:
- Penicillin V.
- Amoxicillin.
- Miconazole (including topical applications).
- Erythromycin.

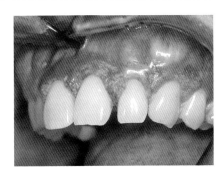

Fig 11-1 Well circumscribed benign osteoma affecting the UL3 region.

- Metronidazole.
- Fluconazole.

If bleeding does not respond to local measures in patients taking warfarin, the use of tranexamic acid is recommended. Tranexamic acid is a non-physiological inhibitor of fibrinolysis and an extremely effective haemostatic agent when used as a mouthwash (5%, 10mls as a rinse for two minutes and then spit out). It can be used four times daily for five to seven days, but avoid food and drink for one hour after rinsing.

Para-Gingival Swellings

Osteomas
Clinical appearance
- Solitary or multiple well-circumscribed swellings (Fig 11-1).
- Bony hard.
- Surface epithelium is intact (no ulceration).

Clinical symptoms
- Painless swelling.

Aetiology
These are benign slow growing tumours of mature bone, usually diagnosed in adult life.

Involvement of non-gingival sites
Multiple osteomas of the jaw are a feature of Gardner's syndrome, a rare autosomal dominant condition. The syndrome also includes:
- Polyposis coli (high incidence of malignant transformation).
- Sebaceous cysts of the skin.

- Multiple fibrous tumours of skin.
- Multiple supernumerary teeth.
- Multiple impacted permanent teeth.

Differential diagnosis
- Torus palatinus or mandibularis.
- Osteoblastoma.
- Osteochondroma (usually in children).
- Ossifying fibroma.
- Ameloblastoma.
- Fibrosarcoma.

Clinical investigation
- Radiology.
- Biopsy.

Management
No treatment unless aesthetic or functional problems have arisen due to the size of the osteoma. In the latter case, surgical re-contouring may be indicated.

Gardner's Syndrome
See above.

Mandibular Tori
Tori are examples of bony 'exostoses', which are benign outgrowths of bone. Normally tori are developmental but they may arise following chronic stimulation as reactive exostoses. The torus palatinus clasically arises in the midline of the palate and the torus mandibularis arises lingual to the mandibular premolar teeth (Fig 11-2). No treatment is indicated unless pre-prosthetic surgery is deemed necessary.

Annular Lesions

Erythema Migrans
Clinical appearance
Erythema migrans may arise in several oral mucosal sites, but usually involves the tongue, where prevalence figures are approximately 2% (Fig 11-3). The term describes red patches, said to look like a map, which vary in size and location, often with a yellow margin surrounding areas of de-papillation.

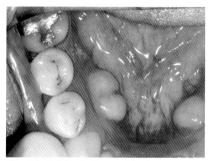

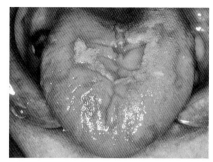

Fig 11-2 Classical mandibular tori.   **Fig 11-3** Erythema migrans.

Clinical symptoms
- Usually asymptomatic.
- Soreness of the tongue, especially with salty or spicy foods.
- Appearance that changes shape and size.

Aetiology
Unknown.

Involvement of non-gingival sites
The tongue dorsum is the most common presenting site, but the palate and buccal mucosa may also be involved.

Differential diagnosis
If the palate is involved it may be confused with:
- Lupus erythematosus.
- Lichen planus.

Clinical investigation
None, the diagnosis is a clinical one

Management
Conservative, avoid irritating foods, and in some cases zinc supplements (200mg, three times daily) may help if taken for two to three months.

Erythema Multiforme
Gingival tissues are typically 'spared' in erythema multiforme and this is one key to differentiating EM lesions from herpes simplex infection. EM is thus not discussed in this text, but is covered in Clerehugh, Tugnait and Chapple (2004, book 17 in this series).

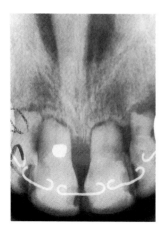

Fig 11-4 Apical third root resorption following adult orthodontic treatment, where the prevalence is higher than in adolescent orthodontics.

Radiological Conditions or Lesions Associated with the Roots

1. Root Resorption

External root resorption can result following a variety of pathological stimuli, the most common being:
• Chronic infection/peri-radicular inflammation.
• Chronic trauma (e.g. excessive orthodontic forces, excessive occlusal forces - Fig 11-4 and 11-5a-d).
• Trauma from hypochlorite irrigation beyond the root canal system.
• Trauma from excessive periodontal instrumentation.
• Impacted or unerupted teeth.
• Cysts (secondary to cyst growth/activity).
• Following tooth luxation and re-implantation.
• Odontogenic tumours (e.g. ameloblastoma).
• Neoplasia (other forms of malignant neoplasia).
• Secondary to radiotherapy of the jaws.

Resorption can also be associated with systemic diseases such as:
• Paget's disease.
• Hypoparathyroidism.
• Hyperparathyroidism.
• Turner's syndrome.
• Calcinosis.
• Gaucher's disease.

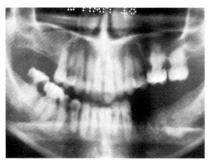

Fig 11-5a Panoramic radiograph of burrowing cervical root resorption in a chronic bruxist who was also a weightlifter.

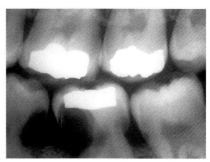

Fig 11-5b Left-sided premolar/molar region in the patient shown in Fig 11-5a prior to extraction of LL56.

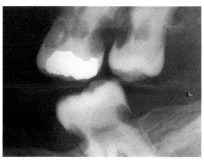

Fig 11-5c Left-sided premolar/molar region in the patient shown in Fig 11-5a post-extraction of LL56. The resorption continued and the LL7 became involved.

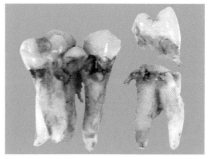

Fig 11-5d The extracted teeth from Fig 11-5b plus an opposing molar.

Fig 11-5e Photomicrograph of cervical dentine resorption from Fig 11-5a-d demonstrating resorption lacunae within the cervical dentine and associated osteoclastic activity.

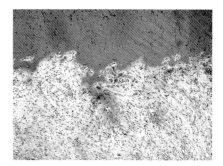

The pathobiology of the resorptive process is not fully understood, but it may affect the apical third of the root (Fig 11-4), the mid-third or the cervical third (Fig 11-5). In the case demonstrated in 11-5a-e it was likely that

227

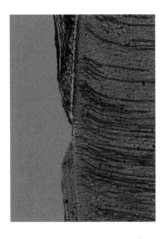

Fig 11-6 Photomicrograph of cementum positioned apical to the CEJ (5-10% of cases).

the cemental layer finished short of the cemento-enamel junction (Fig 11-6) and thus excessive forces on the teeth allowed osteoclastic activity associated with bone remodelling to involve the exposed dentine.

2. Inter- and Peri-radicular Radiolucencies

Systemic Sclerosis (scleroderma)
See Chapter 10.

Periapical Cemental Dysplasia
Periapical cemental dysplasia is a benign condition most commonly affecting the mandibular incisors of post-menopausal females, especially black females. The aetiology is unknown, but the lesions are non-expansile and the teeth vital. Lesions may be solitary or multiple and contain cellular fibrous tissue initially, within which cementum forms. Initially radiolucent (Fig 11-7) and histologically similar to fibrous dysplasia, lesions may gradually become more radio-opaque with time (Fig 11-8) as more cementum is deposited. They can appear like sclerosing osteitis or osteosclerosis, except a fine radiolucent line separates the cementoma from the surrounding bone. No treatment is indicated, as the teeth are vital and the lesions self-limiting.

Lateral Periodontal Cyst (Developmental)
Periodontal cysts are rare and may be:
- Developmental (Fig 11-9).
- Inflammatory (Fig 11-10).

228

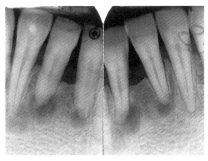

Fig 11-7 Periapical cemental dysplasia in a black female. The lower incisor teeth were vital.

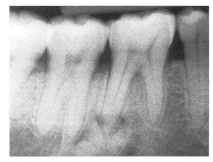

Fig 11-8 Periapical cemental dysplasia with a more radio-opaque appearance due to cementum deposition.

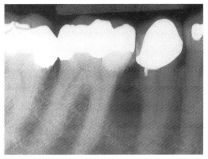

Fig 11-9a A botyroid cyst in a vital tooth pre-surgical enucleation.

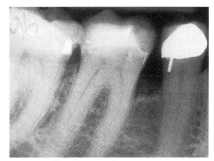

Fig 11-9b The cyst from Fig11-12a 12-months post-enucleation and tissue regeneration using Emdogain™.

Fig 11-10 An inflammatory periodontal cyst affecting UL356 in a 38-year-old female. The cortical plate had perforated palatally and the lesion presented with a clinical depression of the maxillary mucosa.

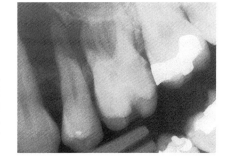

Inflammatory cysts develop following infection of the periodontal or peri-implant tissues and follow a classical course of development from peri- or para-radicular granuloma to cyst formation. They are beyond the scope of

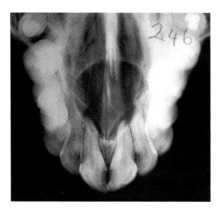

Fig 11-11 A cyst of the incisive (naso-palatine) canal.

this book. However, developmental periodontal cysts are believed to develop in the absence of an inflammatory or infective stimulus from epithelial rests of the embryonic dental lamina. These lesions may be:

• Unilocular lesions.
• Multilocular lesions (Fig 11-9), which are also known as botyroid cysts (after 'bunch of grapes'). Enucleation is indicated as for all periodontal cysts, but botyroid cysts may recur up to 10 years later.

Gingival Cyst

Gingival cysts are rare and present most commonly between the ages of 40–75 years, with 75% of lesions affecting upper canine or pre-molar teeth (Shear, 1985; Wysockie et al, 1980). They may arise mid-way from the cervical margin to the apex, or indeed at the gingival margin where they cause a saucerisation of the alveolar crest. The lesions are soft rather than bony hard (cf lateral periodontal cysts).

Incisive (Naso-palatine) Canal Cyst

Cysts of the nasopalatine or incisive canal are derived from epithelial remains of the nasopalatine duct. Reported prevalence varies between populations (0.1-1.5%) and according to race. Lesions arise apical to the upper incisors. Different parameters are used radiologically to differentiate cystic lesions from normal variations in the canal size. However, most would agree that a cyst should be suspected for lesions >1.0cm diameter where the margin is corticated and for those lesions >1.5cm diameter, cystic change is highly likely (Fig 11-11).

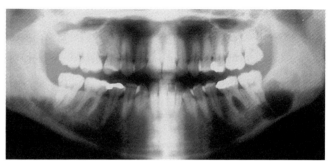

Fig 11-12 An aneurysmal bone cyst.

Patent Nasopalatine Ducts
Patent nasopalatine ducts have been reported to arise clinically either side of the incisive papilla as developmental anomalies. A series of three cases was reported by Chapple and Ord (1990).

Aneurysmal Bone Cyst
These are rare cyst-like lesions filled with sinusoid-like spaces or a single solitary blood-filled space (Fig 11-12).

Squamous Odontogenic Tumour
This is a rare lesion, presenting most often between 20-30 years with an equal male to female ratio. It is often symptomless but can cause tooth migration due to inter-radicular expansion or tooth mobility due to bone resorption. Lesions tend to present as triangular or semi-circular radiolucencies and may have a sclerotic margin. Surgical excision is required.

Ameloblastoma
Ameloblastomas are the most common odontogenic tumours and account for 1% of oral tumours. They are benign but locally invasive lesions that give rise to bone expansion and thinning of the overlying cortex. Eighty per cent are found in the mandible, and of these 70% arise in the molar region, 20% the premolar area and 10% in the lower incisor region. Radiologically the lesions normally appear as multilocular radiolucencies.

The tumours can displace adjacent teeth and cause root resorption. There are three types described:
- Classical – histologically variable, multiple small cysts may fuse to form a large cyst with cuboidal pre-ameloblast cells lining the cyst. Treatment

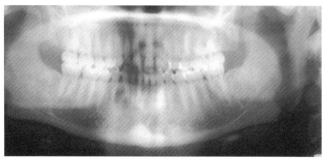

Fig 11-13a A cystic ameloblastoma in a 19-year-old Afro–Caribbean girl. The finding was incidental on a panoramic radiograph (LR45 area), and surgical investigation was indicated due to movement of the roots of the adjacent teeth.

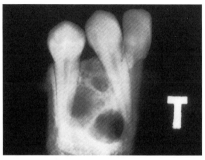

Fig 11-13b The lesion from Fig 11-13a post-block dissection of the affected area.

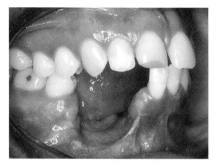

Fig 11-13c The surgical site from Fig 11-13a six months post-resection.

needs to be aggressive and surgical enucleation with a margin of normal bone is advocated (Chapple et al, 1991: Fig 11-13).

- Unicystic – presents in 20-30-year-olds and has a unilocular appearance (hence the name) and responds to curettage or conservative enucleation.
- Peripheral - this is a very rare form of ameloblastoma that affects the soft tissues (without bone involvement).
- Malignant – fortunately extremely rare this form of ameloblastoma does appear to metastasise. However, some believe that rather than true metastasis the tumour is 'seeded' into other tissues by poor surgical technique.

Ameloblastic Fibroma
A rare benign odontogenic tumour that presents in patients <20 years as a slow-growing painless swelling. Radiologically it is a unilocular lesion and

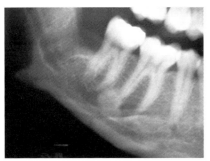 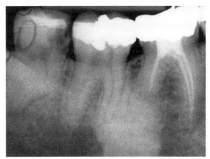

Fig 11-14 Periapical osteoclerosis (sclerosing osteitis) around a tooth, which was also resorbing (mesial root).

Fig 11-15 Condensing osteitis around the distal root apex of LR6, which was vital, but subsequently not filled.

both the epithelial and mesenchymal elements are neoplastic It is, however, non-invasive and therefore it is important to differentiate it from the ameloblastoma, as enucleation can be less radical.

Histiocytosis–X
This condition may present radiologically, and is discussed in Chapter 9 of this text.

3. Inter- and Peri-radicular Radiopacities

Periapical Osteosclerosis
Periapical osteosclerosis refers to localized areas of particularly dense bone, arising in the absence of apparent irritation or infection. It is reported to largely affect posterior teeth with a prevalence as high as 5% (higher in Asians). Radiologically, the marrow space is obliterated (Fig 11-14) and lesions may:
- affect the apical areas of teeth.
- affect inter-radicular regions.
- not be associated with teeth.

No treatment is indicated.

Condensing Osteitis
Pathologists argue that condensing osteitis is the same entity as periapical osteosclerosis. The key difference clinically and radiologically is that condensing osteitis arises adjacent to an area of apical infection (Fig 11-15) and therefore treatment (root canal therapy or extraction) is indicated.

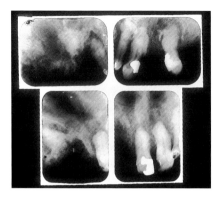

Fig 11-16 Hypercementosis in a patient with Paget's disease.

Hypercementosis

This refers to increased cellular cementum formation normally affecting the apical two-thirds of teeth (Fig 11-16). Causes include:

• Periapical chronic inflammation.
• Occlusal trauma.
• Paget's disease.
• Acromegaly.
• Over-eruption of a tooth with no opposing unit.
• Idiopathic.

Cementomas

Cementomas are benign lesions that are complex to classify as they may arise de-novo or following cementum deposition within other lesions. True cementomas normally affect younger subjects (<25 years) and are more common in males. They are also referred to as benign cementoblastomas and most commonly affect posterior mandibular teeth. Lesions are apical and radiologically appear dense and sclerotic (Fig 11-17). Other lesions within the cementoma group include:

• The gigantiform cementoma (Fig 11-18).
• Periapical cemental dysplasia (see earlier).
• Cementifying fibroma.

Cementicles

These are likely to be dystrophic calcifications within the periodontal ligament rather than true cementomas. They are spherical radiopacities 0.2-0.3mm in diameter and therefore not visible radiographically.

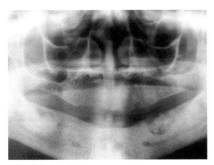 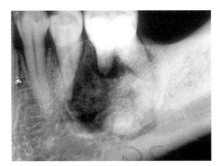

Fig 11-17 Cementoma.   **Fig 11-18** Gigantiform cementoma.

Cementoblastoma
See 'true cementomas'.

Ossifying Fibroma
Also known as 'cementifying fibroma' (see above), these lesions represent variants of the same spectrum of conditions, which also includes 'cemento-ossifying fibroma'. They arise as benign calcifications of fibrous tissue (Fig 11-19) affecting the mandible in 70-90% of cases, with a 5:1 female to male ratio and normally presenting in patients over 40. They are typically solitary lesions that expand in three dimensions and radiologically are well defined radiolucencies within which foci of mineralisation appear. Surgical enucleation is generally relatively simple as lesions are encapsulated. If not encapsulated and removal proves difficult fibrous dysplasia should be suspected (see later).

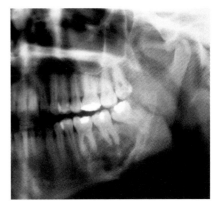

Fig 11-19 Cemento-ossifying fibroma LL67 area. Areas of mineralisation were evident within the body of the radiolucent lesion.

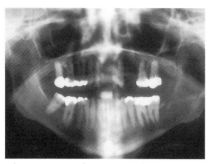

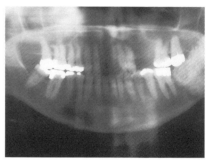

Fig 11-20a Odontogenic keratocyst of the mandible pre-marsupialisation in a 40-year-old female.

Fig 11-20b The keratocyst from Fig 11-20a immediately post-surgery and packing.

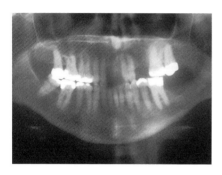

Fig 11-20c The cyst from Fig11-20a four months post-surgery.

4. Radiolucent Lesions – Well Circumscribed Radiolucencies

Odontogenic Keratocyst
Radiological appearance
Radiological appearances vary:
- Well-circumscribed radiolucent lesion within the medullary space.
- Unilocular or multilocular appearances may arise.
- Most commonly affect mandible (65-85%). Molar/ramus region accounts for about 50%.
- Cysts become large and fill entire ramus with time (Fig 11-20).
- Perforations of the cortical plate may be seen.
- Margins become sclerotic with time.
- Cyst cavity becomes 'foggy' with time due to keratin deposition.
- Root resorption is NOT characteristic.
- May arise bilaterally in young patients (<10 years) as part of the Gorlin-Goltz syndrome.

236

Clinical symptoms
Cysts arise in the second and third decade, and symptoms are rare because cysts permeate the mandible in an antero-posterior direction, becoming extremely large before detection. Often they are an incidental radiographic finding.

Aetiology and involvement of non-gingival sites
Odontogenic keratocysts (OKC's) are believed to develop from remnants of the embryonic dental lamina from which the tooth germ develops; the term 'primordial cyst' is therefore also applied to the same lesions.

Differential diagnosis
- Dentigerous cyst.
- Lateral periodontal cyst.
- Inflammatory/radicular cyst associated with tooth apex.
- Residual cyst.
- Ameloblastoma.
- Odontogenic fibroma.
- Odontogenic myxoma.
- Central giant cell granuloma.
- Aneurysmal bone cyst.
- Brown tumour (of hyperparathyroidism).

Clinical investigation
- Additional radiographic views to assess expansion/extent within bone:
  - Lateral oblique view of mandible.
  - True occlusal view (bucco-lingual extent).
  - Postero-anterior view focussed on jaws.
  - CT scan.
- Broad needle aspirate will yield a thick yellow/brown cheese-like material comprising keratin squames and low protein levels (<40g/L).
- Incisional biopsy to include bone and any putative lining epithelium.

Management
OKCs are notoriously difficult to remove because:
- The lining fibrous capsule is friable and thin and easily torn/left behind during enucleation.
- There are frequently 'daughter cysts' (satellite cysts) beyond the main lesion.
- Projections of the main cyst may be missed at surgery.

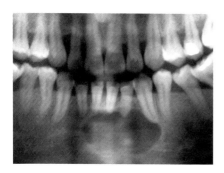

Fig 11-21 An inflammatory apical cyst associated with non-vital LL12.

Due to difficulties with complete enucleation, recurrence rates of between 12-63% are reported and recurrence may take up to 25 years. The case in Fig 11-20a was therefore marsupialised and packed with ribbon gauze soaked in 'Whitehead's varnish'. The pack was replaced every few weeks until bone filled the defect from the mandibular base. This approach reduced the risk of manbibular fracture at surgery and also the risk of recurrence (Fig 11-20b and c).

Inflammatory Cyst
Inflammatory cysts are very common around tooth apices where:
- A non-vital pulp has become infected.
- A root is retained (and infected).
- A root canal filling has failed.
- A root has fractured.
- There is a root perforation or infected lateral canal.
- A retrograde root filling has failed to eliminate pathology.

Lesions are well circumscribed radiolucencies (Fig 11-21) and with time the margin can become corticated. Similar lesions may also arise around implants (Fig 11-22a-c).

Neural Sheath Tumours
Neural sheath tumours are rare benign lesions which may present from birth to 70yrs as intra-osseous radiolucencies. Clinical symptoms include:
- Dysasthesia/parasthesia.
- Burning sensation.
- Pain.

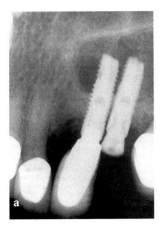
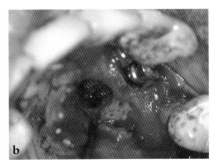
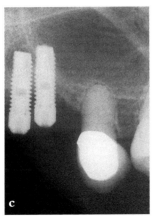

Fig 11-22a Inflammatory peri-implant cyst pre-surgical enucleation. The cyst communicated with the maxillary antrum.

Fig 11-22b The cyst in Fig 11-22a at the time of surgery. The cyst cavity was packed with BioOss™ and covered with a Bioguide™ membrane for 12 months.

Fig 11-22c The healed site from Fig 11-22b 12 months post-surgery with a small residual scar around the mesial implant.

Broadly there are several lesions within this group:
- Neurilemmoma – well encapsulated lesions.
- Schwannoma – can arise peripherally within soft tissue (Fig 11-23).
- Neurofibroma – solitary lesions which are more likely to recur as less well encapsulated (Chapter 5 - Fig 5-13).
- Neurofibromatosis – multiple neurofibromas may arise as part of von Recklinghausen's neurofibromatosis, characterised by multiple lesions of the skin, which are hamartomas rather than true neoplasms (see Chapter 7).

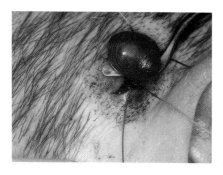

Fig 11-23 An 'Ancient Schwannoma' at enucleation. It was well encapsulated and comprised degenerative nerve tissue.

Multi-locular Radiolucencies

Odontogenic Keratocyst and Gorlin-Goltz Syndrome

OKC's have been discussed previously. They may arise as multiple lesions in the autosomal dominantly-inherited Gorlin-Goltz syndrome, which is characterised by:

- Multiple OKCs of the jaws.
- Multiple skin basal cell carcinomas.
- Rib/vertebral deformity.
- Bossing of the frontal and temporal bones of the skull.
- Calcifications of the falx cerebri.

Botyroid Cyst

See above.

Ameloblastoma

See above.

Odontogenic Myxoma

The odontogenic fibroma, may arise centrally or peripherally, where it is almost identical to the fibrous epulis (Chapter 5). They are however extremely rare and not discussed further (see Soames and Southam, 1993). The odontogenic myxoma is more common and normally presents as a multilocular lesion (though it may be unilocular) radiographically. It is less well-defined than the odontogenic fibroma and locally invasive, hence enucleation is problematic.

Giant Cell Tumour of Bone

Giant cell lesions of the jaws are histologically the same, but true giant cell tumours of the jaws (osteoclastoma), unlike central giant cell granulomas,

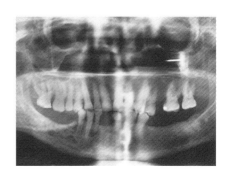

Fig 11-24 Osteomyelitis affecting LR234, with characteristic 'moth-eaten' appearance.

are destructive/aggressive lesions that metastasise and behave more like true sarcomas. Fortunately, true giant cell tumours of the jaws are extremely rare.

Aneurysmal Bone Cyst
These lesions may be uni- or multilocular and tend to affect the posterior mandible. They comprise blood filled spaces and largely arise secondary to other bone pathology, such as giant cell granulomas.

Arterio-venous Malformations (AVMs)
AVMs are discussed in Chapter 3.

Sturge Weber Syndrome
Sturge Weber syndrome discussed in Chapter 4.

Cherubism
Also known as familial fibrous dysplasia, cherubism is an autosomal domi-nant-inherited disorder that presents between two to five years of age. Multi-locular cystic lesions appear in the mandible and maxilla, but the condition usually regresses by the age of 20 years. Other features include:
- Bilateral swelling of the cheeks (so-called 'cherubic' appearance) usually affecting the mandibular angles and posterior maxillary sinuses.
- 'Cafe au lait' pigmentation of skin.
- Multiple unerupted or ectopic teeth.
- Accelerated deciduous tooth resorption.

Ossifying Fibroma
A slow-growing and well-encapsulated benign tumour of fibrous tissue, within which ossification or cementification may occur. Usually affects chil-dren and adolescents, and its encapsulation helps distinguish it from fibrous dysplasia. Biopsy is essential for histological diagnosis.

241

Poorly Defined Radiolucent Lesions

Osteomyelitis
Osteomyelitis is inflammation of the bone marrow and tends to arise in the jaws following deep-seated odontogenic infection in debilitated or immuno-suppressed patients or those with limited blood supply to the mandible. Pre-disposing conditions include:
- Diabetes mellitus.
- Paget's disease.
- Osteopetrosis.
- Trauma to the mandible (e.g. fracture).
- Long-standing odontogenic infection.
- Radiotherapy to the jaws.

Soames and Southam (1993) classify osteomyelitis into:
- Suppurative (acute or chronic).
- Chronic sclerosing (focal or diffuse).
- Special types
  - radiation
  - chemical
  - osteomyelitis of the newborn.

Associated mainly with gram – ve organisms, the inflammation and infec-tion give rise to compromised local blood flow and areas of bone necrosis develop (bone sequestra). The inflammation/infection spreads throughout the bone marrow and eventually the periosteal blood supply is compromised. Radiologically a 'moth-eaten' appearance is ascribed (Fig 11-24) to the bone as radiolucent areas have a poorly defined margin and bone sequestra within the lesion appear radiopaque. Treatment is aggressive and involves surgical curettage, removal of sequestra and systemic antibiotics.

Osteoradionecrosis
This is a form of bone necrosis that arises following radiotherapy to the jaws. The radiotherapy causes an endarteritis obliterans and loss of blood supply to areas of bone, which necroses and is more susceptible to infection. This may ultimately give rise to mandibular fracture (Millett et al, 1990).

Intraosseous Carcinoma
True intraosseous carcinomas are extremely rare and usually arise in chil-dren.

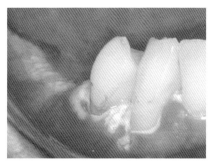 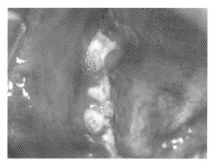

Fig 11-25a Keratosis associated with underlying carcinoma cuniculatum of the gingivae.

Fig 11-25b The same lesion as Fig 11-25a at a later stage and after a third biopsy.

Gingival Carcinoma
- Squamous cell carcinoma (see Chapter 8).
- Carcinoma cuniculatum (Fig 11-25) is a rare variant of squamous cell carcinoma, which is extremely slow growing but invades bone and surrounding tissue. It may take several years to develop and can present as keratosis with varying degrees of ulceration and/or suppuration, due to infection of underlying necrotic bone. Heasman et al (2005) presented a case in a 44-year-old female that was only diagnosed following a deep biopsy of bone. Lesions may be mistakenly diagnosed as osteomyelitis. Metastasis to regional lymph nodes is rare.

Ameloblastic Carcinoma
This lesion is the same as a malignant ameloblastoma (see earlier).

Radiolucent Lesions as Presentations of Systemic Disease

Histiocytosis–X
See Chapter 9.

Multiple Myeloma
Myeloma is a malignant proliferation of a clone of immunoglobulin producing plasma cells which may arise as:
- Solitary plasmacytoma (a solitary myeloma – very rare).
- Multiple myeloma (normally a disseminated disease of poor prognosis).

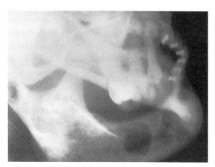

Fig 11-26 Multipe myeloma.

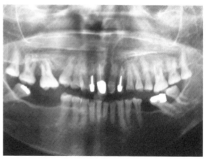

Fig 11-27 Prominent trabeculation and marrow hyperplasia (and osteopaenia) secondary to thalassaemia. The maxillary antrum is also full of trabecular bone as the body attempts to synthesise more red blood cells.

Excess production of a monoclonal immunoglobulin is also referred to as a 'monoclonal gammopathy'. These are often benign but 10% may become malignant with time and monitoring is therefore important. With malignant myeloma the light chains of the immunoglobulin are small enough to be excreted through the kidney and appear in urine as 'Bence-Jones protein'. The cranial bones and jaws can be affected with multiple 'punched out' osteolytic lesions (Fig 11-26) and clinical signs/symptoms may include:
- Bone pain.
- Renal failure.
- Anaemia (oral ulceration secondary to bone marrow suppression).
- Recalcitrant infections of the jaws.
- Unusual or exaggerated bleeding post-periodontal or surgical therapy.
- Macroglossia (secondary to amyloid deposition within the tongue).

Non-Hodgkins Lymphoma (see Chapter 8)
A malignant lymphoma affecting young adults, which may present as:
- Painless enlargement of lymph nodes.
- Paraesthesia/anaesthesia.
- Soft swelling around fauces or maxillary gingivae.
- Ulceration around tonsillar region.
- Mobility of teeth with associated swelling.

The lymphomas are classified histologically, with diffuse lesions having a poorer prognosis than focal (follicular) lesions. Broadly lesions are either:

- High grade (poor prognosis but often respond well to chemotherapy).
- Low grade (good prognosis).

Underlying risk factors include:
- Immunosuppression.
- AIDS.
- Some autoimmune diseases (e.g. Sjögrens syndrome).

Leukaemia
See earlier.

Generalised Radiolucencies

Hypophosphatasia
This condition is discussed in Chapter 10.

Hyperparathyroidism
This condition results in excess parathyroid hormone (PTH) and may be primary in nature or secondary to chronic hypocalcaemia. Primary hyperparathyroidism may arise due to lesions affecting the parathyroid glands, e.g:
- Benign hyperplasia.
- Adenoma.
- Adencarcinoma.

PTH causes calcium retention and achieves this by increasing intestinal absorption and renal resorption, but also by increasing osteoclastic activity in bone. The latter can give rise to osteolytic lesions called 'brown tumours' (due to deposition of haemosiderin), where fibrous tissue replaces mineralised bone. The latter contain giant cells and are histologically identical to giant cell tumours/granulomas of bone (see earlier).

Sickle Cell Anaemia
Sickle cell anaemia affects 1 in 500 black people and radiologically can cause marrow hyperplasia and prominent trabeculation. Thalassaemia may cause similar radiological changes (Fig 11-27).

5. Radiolucent Lesions with Radiopacities

Periapical Cemental Dysplasia
See earlier.

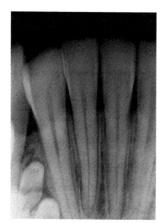

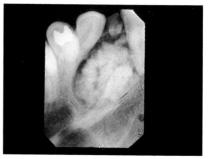

Fig 11-29 Complex odontome.

Fig 11-28 Compound odontome.

Calcifying Odontogenic Cyst

These are not true cysts and regarded by most as odontogenic tumours. They arise as slow growing enlargements of the gingivae or adjacent alveolar mucosa from the pre-molar region forwards. They may appear as unilocular or multilocular radiolucencies, within which there is calcification of enlarged keratinocytes called 'Ghost cells'. Enucleation is usually successful.

Calcifying Epithelial Odontogenic Tumour (CEOT)

Also referred to as Pindborg's tumour, the CEOT is a benign but locally invasive odontogenic tumour of epithelial origin. The lesion appears as an irregular radiolucency in which radiopaque areas develop following calcification.

Adenomatoid Odontogenic Tumour

This tumour is benign and well-encapsulated, arising in the anterior maxilla. It appears as a well-defined radiolucency, within which calcification may occur. It can be enucleated simply and should be differentiated from an ameloblastoma for this reason.

Odontomes

Odontomes are hamartomatous lesions of dental tissues that by definition contain enamel and dentine. They vary in shape and size but compound (Fig 11-28) and complex (Fig 11-29) odontomes are most likely to present as incidental radiological findings.

246

6. Radiopaque Lesions – Focal Radiopacities

Osteoma
See earlier.

Osteosarcoma
This is the most common malignant primary bone tumour, but is fortunately very rare in the jaws. It presents radiologically as an irregular radiolucency within which varying degrees of neoplastic bone may appear as radiopaque areas. When the tumour perforates the cortical plate it lifts the periosteum and trabeculae of bone span out at 90° to the cortex, giving the characteristic 'sun-ray spicule' appearance, although this is an unusual finding in the jaws.

Generalised Radiopacities

Gardner's Syndrome
See above.

Sclerosing Osteomyelitis
See earlier.

Fibrous Dysplasia
This is a non-heritable developmental disorder that may affect the mandible or maxilla and presents during childhood or adolescence (i.e. during active skeletal development), normally becoming quiescent in adulthood. It presents as a slow growing, painless enlargement of the posterior maxilla or mandible, which is often unilateral (unlike Cherubism) and causes facial asymmetry. Two forms are described:
• Monostotic (localised).
• Polyostotic (several bones involved).

The aetiology is unknown and management usually involves cosmetic debulking surgery (Fig 11–30).

Albright's Syndrome
This syndrome involves:
• Polyostotic fibrous dysplasia.
• 'Café au lait' pigmentation of skin and oral mucosa.
• Precocious puberty in females.

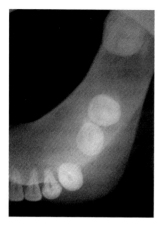

Fig 11-30 Fibrous dysplasia.

Paget's Disease of Bone

Thought to have a viral aetiology (paramyxovirus), Paget's disease is a chronic deforming bone disease in which bone remodelling is chaotic. Progressive enlargement of the facial and skull bones arises, as do similar changes in the peripheral skeleton. Encroachment on cranial nerve fossae and canals can give rise to:

- Deafness.
- Visual abnormalities.
- Facial palsy.
- Motor defects.

As the bones thicken, secondary problems arise from intermittent cycles of bone resorption and deposition. These include:

- Pathological fractures.
- Disrupted occlusion.
- Hypercementosis.
- Ankylosis.
- Difficult extractions (due to the above).
- Post-extraction haemorrhage.
- Post-extraction infections.
- Root resorption.

Radiologically, areas of mixed osteosclerosis and osteoporosis give rise to a so-called 'cotton wool' appearance to bone (Fig 11-31).

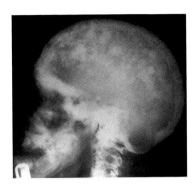

Fig 11-31 Paget's disease of bone.

Osteopetrosis

Also called Albers-Schonberg disease (or marble bone disease) osteopetrosis is a defect of osteoclast activity that leads to excess bone deposition. The dense bone is prone to fracture and anaemia may arise as a secondary complication of marrow obliteration. Benign and malignant forms are described, the former presenting later in life whereas the latter is fatal in childhood. Radiologically bone is extremely dense and teeth may appear to disappear!

Hyperostosis

Two forms are described:
- Endosteal (autosomal recessive).
- Infantile cortical (idiopathic).

The condition is beyond the scope of this book, but is included because it may be a differential diagnosis for thickened and sclerotic bone changes seen on radiographs of the skull and facial bones.

Further Reading

Baxter AM, Roberts A, Shaw L, Chapple ILC. Localised scleroderma in a 12-year-old girl presenting as gingival recession. A case report and literature review. Dental Update 2001;28:458-462.

Chapple IL, Ord RA. Three cases of patent nasopalatine canals: case reports and a review of the literature. Oral Surgery, Oral Medicine, Oral Pathology 1990;69:554-558.

Chapple ILC, Manogue M. Management of recurrent follicular ameloblastoma. Dental Update 1991;18:309-312.

Chapple ILC, Thorpe GHG, Smith JM et al. Hypophosphatasia: a family study involving a case diagnosed from gingival crevicular fluid. Journal of Clinical Periodontology 1992;21:426-431.

Chapple ILC. Hypophosphatasia: dental aspects and mode of inheritance. Journal of Clinical Periodontology 1993;20:615-622.

Chapple I L C, Saxby M S, Murray J. Gingival haemorrhage, myelodysplastic syndromes and acute myeloid leukaemia. Journal of Periodontology 1999;70:1247-1253.

Devani P, Lavery K M, Howell C J T. 1998. Dental Extractions in Patients on Warfarin: Is Alteration of Anticoagulant Regime Necessary? British Journal of Oral and Maxillofacial Surgery 36: 107-111.

Gaspar, Brenner, Ardekian, Peled, Laufer. 1997. Use of Tranexamic Acid Mouthwash to Prevent Post-Operative Bleeding in Oral Surgery Patients on Oral Anticoagulant Medication. Quintessence International, 28: 375-379.

Diagnostic Imaging of the Jaws. 1995. Langlais R.P., Langland O.E. & Nortjé C.J. (Eds). Williams and Wilkins. IBSN: 0-683-04809-0.
Drugs Diseases and the Periodontium. 1992. Seymour R.A. & Heasman P.H. (Eds). Oxford Medical Publications. ISBN: 0-19-261992-6.

Heasman P A, Smith D G, Martin I, Soames J. 2005. Carcinoma cuniculatum presenting as a gingival lesion. PERIO in Practice Today (in press).

Millet D T, Chapple I L C, Hirschman P, Corrigan M. 1990. Septic osteoradionecrosis of the mandible associated with pathological fracture: report of two cases. Journal of Clinical Radiology, 41: 408-410.

Oral Pathology (2nd Edition). 1993. Soames J. V. & Southam J. C. (Eds). Oxford Medical Publications. ISBN:0 19 2622153.

Shear M. Cysts of the jaws: recent advances. 1985. Journal of Oral Pathology, 14: 43.

Souto J C, Oliver A et al. 1996. Oral Surgery in Anticoagulated Patients without Reducing the Dose of Oral Anticoagulant: A Prospective Randomised Study. Journal of Oral and Maxillofacial Surgery 54: 27-32.

Wahl M J. 2000. Myths of Dental Surgery in Patients Receiving Anticoagulant Therapy. Journal of the American Dental Association 131: 77-81.

Wysocki G P, Brannon R B, Gardner D C, Sapp P. 1980. Histogenesis of the lateral periodontal cyst and gingival cyst of the adult. Oral Surgery, Oral Medicine, Oral Pathology, 50: 327.

Index

von Recklinghausen's disease 93

von-Willebrand factor
 deficiency 221

W

Wegener's granulomatosis 125

White sponge naevus of
 Cannon 41, 49

Wiskott Aldrich
 syndrome 158, 196, 205

X

Xerostomia 10, 206

Z

Zidovudine 18

Endodontics, Editor: John M Whitworth

    Rational Root Canal Treatment in Practice   available
    Managing Endodontic Failure in Practice   available
    Restoring Endodontically Treated Teeth   Autumn 2006

Prosthodontics, Editor: P Finbarr Allen

    Teeth for Life for Older Adults   available
    Complete Dentures – from Planning to Problem Solving   available
    Removable Partial Dentures   available
    Fixed Prosthodontics in Dental Practice   available
    Occlusion: A Theoretical and Team Approach   Autumn 2006

Operative Dentistry, Editor: Paul A Brunton

    Decision-Making in Operative Dentistry   available
    Aesthetic Dentistry   available
    Communicating in Dental Practice   available
    Indirect Restorations   Summer 2006
    Choosing and Using Dental Materials   Autumn 2006

Paediatric Dentistry/Orthodontics, Editor: Marie Therese Hosey

    Child Taming: How to Cope with Children in Dental Practice available
    Paediatric Cariology   available
    Treatment Planning for the Developing Dentition   available
    Managing Dental Trauma in Practice   available

General Dentistry and Practice Management, Editor: Raj Rattan

    The Business of Dentistry   available
    Risk Management   available
    Quality Matters: From Clinical Care to Customer Service   Summer 2006
    Practice Management for the Dental Team   Autumn 2006
    Dental Practice Design   Autumn 2006
    Handling Complaint in Dental Practice   Autumn 2006

Dental Team, Editor: Mabel Slater

    Team Players in Dentistry   Autumn 2006

Quintessence Publishing Co. Ltd., London

Quintessentials for General Dental Practitioners Series

in 50 volumes

Editor-in-Chief: Professor Nairn H F Wilson

General Dentistry, Editor: Nairn Wilson

Implantology in General Dental Practice	available
Culturally Sensitive Oral Healthcare	available
Dental Erosion	available
Managing Orofacial Pain in Practice	Autumn 2006
Dental Bleaching	Autumn 2006
Special Care Dentistry	Autumn 2006
Infection Control for the Dental Team	Spring 2007
Therapeutics and Medical Emergencies in the Everyday Clinical Practice of Dentistry	Spring 2007

Oral Surgery and Oral Medicine, Editor: John G Meechan

Practical Dental Local Anaesthesia	available
Practical Oral Medicine	available
Practical Conscious Sedation	available
Minor Oral Surgery in Dental Practice	available

Imaging, Editor: Keith Horner

Interpreting Dental Radiographs	available
Panoramic Radiology	available
Twenty-first Century Dental Imaging	Autumn 2006

Periodontology, Editor: Iain L C Chapple

Understanding Periodontal Diseases: Assessment and Diagnostic Procedures in Practice	available
Decision-Making for the Periodontal Team	available
Successful Periodontal Therapy – A Non-Surgical Approach	available
Periodontal Management of Children, Adolescents and Young Adults	available
Periodontal Medicine: A Window on the Body	available